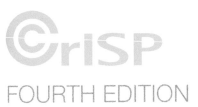

CriSP

FOURTH EDITION

Care of the Critically Ill
Surgical Patient®

Faculty Handbook

Edited by
Danny Bryden and John Jameson

First published in Great Britain in 1999 by the Royal College of Surgeons of England
Second edition 2003
Third edition 2010
This fourth edition published in 2017 by
The Royal College of Surgeons of England
 35-43 Lincoln's Inn Fields, London, WC2A 3PE

www.rcseng.ac.uk

Whilst the advice and information in this book are believed to be true and accurate at the date of going to press, neither the author[s] nor the publisher can accept any legal responsibility or liability for any errors or omissions that may be made. In particular (but without limiting the generality of the preceding disclaimer) every effort has been made to check drug dosages; however, it is still possible that errors have been missed. Furthermore, dosage schedules are constantly being revised and new side-effects recognized. For these reasons the reader is strongly urged to consult the drug companies' printed instructions before administering any of the drugs recommended in this book.

British Library Cataloguing in Publication Data

A catalogue record for this book is available from the British Library

Library of Congress Cataloging-in-Publication Data

A catalogue record for this book is available from the Library of Congress

ISBN 978-1-904096-33-7

Typeset by Prepress Projects Ltd

Contents

Contents

Using the 4th edition materials

This edition includes a coding system to help you link course materials with book chapters.

Each item of course material has an index number, which links to sections in this manual. Such as:

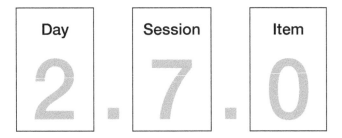

Day	Session	Item
2	. 7	. 0

In this example, document 2.7.0 is the first item you'll need to support session 7 on the second day of the course, in this case a history chart in the first moulage.

They are also colour coded to make it easy to link chapters in the manual to the loose materials.

Two-day CCrISP course programme: resources and timing

Resource number	Time		Title
	Start	**Finish**	
Day One			
	8:00 am	8:30 am	Registration/Faculty Meeting
1.0	8:30 am	8:40 am	Welcome and Introductions
1.1	8:40 am	9:10 am	Introduction to CCrISP and assessment of the critically ill surgical patient
1.2	9:10 am	9:30 am	Demonstration: Patient Assessment
	9:30 am	10:50 am	Practical skills rotation – Assessment of the critically ill surgical patient (20 minutes each)
1.3			Scenario A: Stridor
1.4			Scenario B: Haemothorax/rib fracture
1.5			Scenario C: Sepsis
1.6			Scenario D: Narcotised patient
	10:50 am	11:05 am	Break
	11:05 am	12:45 pm	Small group sessions (25 minutes each)
1.7			Respiratory Failure
1.8			Tracheostomy management
1.9			Wound Care
1.10			Stoma care
	12:45 pm	1:15 pm	Lunch
	1:15 pm	4:30 pm	Small group sessions (45 minutes each)
1.11			Perioperative cardiac disorder
1.12			Cardiovascular manipulation in shock

	2:45 pm	3:00 pm	Break (rotation continues after break)
1.13			Professional skills
1.14			Acute Kidney Injury
1.15	4:30 pm	5:30 pm	Nutrition
	5:30 pm		Faculty meeting
Day Two			
	7:50 am	8:00 am	Registration
	8:00 am	11:15 am	Small group sessions (45 minutes each)
2.0			The Unwell Surgical Patient
2.1			Ward Dilemmas
	9:30 am	9:45 am	Break (rotation continues after break)
2.2			Pain Management
2.3			Respiratory Care and Chest Imaging
2.4	11:15 am	11:30 am	Course Summary
2.5	11:30 am	12:10 pm	Demonstration Patient Assessment video
	12:10 pm	1:00 pm	Lunch
	1:00 pm	4:00 pm	Moulage/Virtual Ward Round rotation
2.6, 2.7 or 2.8			Moulage (1st of 3 choices)
2.6, 2.7 or 2.8			Moulage (2nd of 3 choices)
Staggered break between the sessions. Candidates should not mix between the sessions.			
	2:15 pm	2:30 pm	Break (for candidates doing Virtual Ward Round first)
	2:30 pm	2:45 pm	Break (for candidates doing Moulages first)
2.9			Virtual Ward Round
	4:00 pm	4:30 pm	Candidate break/Faculty meeting
	4:30 pm	4:45 pm	Candidate feedback

Foreword

Since its introduction in January 1996, the Care of the Critically Ill Surgical Patient (CCrISP) course of The Royal College of Surgeons of England has expanded to become an integral part of the early years of surgical training. Its success has led it to be taught in over 44 centres throughout the UK and also in Ireland, Italy, Singapore, Malaysia and Australasia.

The CCrISP course teaching materials have been in use since 2010 and a review was timely. John Jameson and Danny Bryden are to be congratulated for their hard work in producing this 4th edition. It promises to be a successful and valuable update. The revisions have been made by a multidisciplinary working group after canvassing opinion from many CCrISP instructors. This consensus process has produced course documents based on established mainstream medical practice and which should be uncontroversial for participants to use to treat patients in any hospital or to discuss in any examination. One particularly striking and useful change is the cross-referencing to early warning scores. This should help our young colleagues determine how ill patients are as well to institute structured acute care in real-life practice. The CCrISP system of assessment continues to underpin the course but the new and more varied clinical cases should illustrate key points more effectively.

This 4th edition features a new 2-day structure and should fit better with modern time constraints. Piloting of the modified course has certainly produced very positive feedback. This faculty handbook details the individual components of the course and indicates ways to teach each session. The aim has been to make it as easy as possible for you to prepare for teaching on the CCrISP course with a simplified set of course materials. That should save you time and let you concentrate on making the course as realistic and valuable a clinical experience for candidates as it can be.

It is particularly appropriate to acknowledge the generous support of the Hillsborough Trust, which sponsored the original development of the CCrISP programme in memory of the 96 fans who died in the stadium tragedy. It is also poignant to acknowledge the unstinting financial support of Jane and Leon Grant over many years given Jane's sad passing. As a former survivor of surgical critical illness Jane channelled her desire for better care standards with both charm and determination.

The success of CCrISP is based on its ability to match the perceived needs of trainees and patients. Fundamental to this success is the ability, enthusiasm and commitment that you, the instructors, bring to the course wherever it is run. We hope you enjoy teaching with the new material and that you find it a useful vehicle for passing on your clinical experience in a structured way. With pressure from greater external scrutiny of medical practice and a diminished team structure to support them, the help that the CCrISP course gives young trainees and their patients remains very important.

Thank you very much for your continued support, which makes a huge difference to the success of the course.

Iain D Anderson MBE MD FRCS(Eng, Edin, Glas) FRACS(Hon)

4th edition contributors

Editors

Dr Daniele Bryden	MB ChB, FRCA, FFICM, LLB(Hons), MML	Consultant in Intensive Care Medicine and Anaesthesia, Sheffield Teaching Hospitals NHS Foundation Trust, Sheffield, England
Mr John S Jameson	MA(Cantab), MB BS, FRCS, MD	Consultant Colorectal Surgeon, University Hospitals of Leicester NHS Trust, Leicester General Hospital, Leicester, England

Steering group members

Mr Brian Johnson	MD, FRCS	Consultant Vascular Surgeon, Hull Royal Infirmary, Kingston upon Hull, England
Dr Jon Walton	MBChB, MRCP, FRCA DipICM	Consultant in Critical Care Medicine and Anaesthesia, Freeman Hospital, Newcastle upon Tyne, England
Dr Sarah Gillis	FRCA, FFICM	Consultant Anaesthetist with an interest in ICM, Whittington Hospital, London, England
Mr Andrew Kordowicz	MA, MB, BChir, MEd, MRCS	Specialist Registrar Vascular Surgery, Hull Royal Infirmary, Kingston upon Hull, England
Dr Joseph F Cosgrove	MB BS, FRCA, FFICM	Consultant in Anaesthesia and Intensive Care Medicine, Freeman Hospital, Newcastle upon Tyne, England
Dr Philip Buckley	MBChB, FRCA	Consultant Anaesthetist, Hull & East Yorkshire Hospitals NHS Trust, Kingston upon Hull, England
Mr Ben Lindsey	FRCS	Consultant Vascular and Renal Transplant Surgeon, The Royal Free London NHS Foundation Trust, London, England

Contributors

Dr Karen Kerr	MBChB FRCA	Consultant Anaesthetist, Sheffield Teaching Hospitals NHS Foundation Trust, Sheffield, England
Dr Mike Fried	BSc (Hons), MB BS, MRCGP, FRCA, FFARCSI	Consultant in Anaesthesia and Critical Care Medicine, St John's Hospital, Livingston, Scotland
Mr Marius Berman	MD, FRCS (CTh)	Consultant Cardiothoracic and Transplant Surgeon, Papworth Hospital, Cambridge, England
Dr Thanthullu Vasu	MB BS, MD, DNB, FRCA, FFPMRCA, Dip Pain Mgt	Consultant and Head of Pain Service, University Hospitals of Leicester NHS Trust, Leicester, England
Dr Shyam Balasubramanian	MBBS MD MSc FRCA FFPMRCA	Consultant in Pain Medicine and Anaesthesia, University Hospitals of Coventry and Warwickshire, NHS Trust, Coventry, England
Dr Mathew V Patteril	MD DA FRCA DipClinEdu(RCS)	Consultant Cardiothoracic Anaesthetist, Department of Anaesthesia, Critical Care and Pain Management, University Hospitals of Coventry and Warwickshire NHS Trust, Coventry, England
Dr Simon Gabe	MD, MSc, MBBS, BSc(Hons), FRCP	Consultant Gastroenterologist & Honorary Senior Lecturer and Co-Chair of the Lennard-Jones Intestinal Failure Unit, St Mark's Hospital, Harrow, England
Dr Deborah Kerr	MCEM, FRCA	Advanced ICM trainee, Sheffield Teaching Hospitals NHS Foundation Trust, Sheffield, England
Dr Arunan Yogasundaram	FRCA	Critical Care Fellow, Alfred Hospital, Melbourne, Australia

Pilot faculty

Mr Paul Froggatt

Mr Ashar Wadoodi

Mr Louis Fligelstone

Mr Andrew Lee

Miss Sarah Thommaset

Contributors to previous editions

Contributors to the 3rd edition

Mr Ian Loftus	FRCS
Mr Iain Anderson	FRCS
Dr Daniele Bryden	FRCA
Mr Francis Calder	FRCSEd
Dr Joe Cosgrove	FRCA
Dr Sarah Gillis	FRCA
Dr Jonathan Goodall	FRCA
Mr John Jameson	FRCS
Mr Brian Johnson	FRCS
Mr Keith Jones	FRCS
Dr Philip Newman	FRCA
Dr Declan O'Brian	FRCA
Professor Rob Sayers	FRCS
Mr Mark Taylor	FRCS

Contributors to the 2nd edition

Mr G L Carlson

Dr M Hunter

Dr B Riley

Professor B J Rowlands

Dr G B Smith

Professor M M Thompson

Contributors to the 1st edition

Dr T N Appleyard

Professor K Fearon

Mr D R Griffin

Professor D J Leaper

Dr G Ramsay

Mr R C G Russell

Professor J M Ryan

Dr A I K Short

Dr S W Turner

Dr R G Wheatley

Acknowledgements

Peter Loader MSc
Senior Project Manager
Royal College of Surgeons of England

Course objectives

- Develop the theoretical basis and practical skills necessary to manage the critically ill surgical patient.

- Be able to assess critically ill patients accurately and appreciate the value of using a system of assessment.

- Understand the subtlety and variety of presentation of critical illness and the methods available for improving detection.

- Appreciate that complications tend to occur in a cascade and realise that prevention of complications is fundamental to a successful outcome.

- Be aware of multidisciplinary teamworking and understand how members of the team interact to support the patient, who is at the centre of the process.

- Be aware of the importance of the lead role the surgeon needs to assume in coordinating this care and making decisions as necessary.

- Understand the importance of a plan of action in order to achieve clinical progress, accurate diagnosis and early definitive treatment.

- Be able to ensure that the plan of action is carried out accurately and in a timely manner and that it is communicated to all the relevant people, including the patient and relatives.

- Ensure that the assessment, decision-making process and communication are accurately and adequately documented in the patient's case notes.

- Understand the requirements of the patient and his or her relatives during critical illness and be able to inform, involve and support the patient and relatives appropriately.

- An aide-memoire for success is to:

    - ACCEPT responsibility for patient management.

    - ADOPT a systematic approach to patient assessment.

    - APPRECIATE that complications tend to cascade rapidly.

    - ANTICIPATE and prevent complications with simple, timely actions.

    - APPLY effective communication skills to facilitate patient care.

    - ASK for appropriate assistance in a timely manner.

The CCrISP system of assessment

Immediate management
Airway | Breathing | Circulation | Dysfunction of CNS | Exposure

Full patient assessment
Chart review | History and systematic examination | Available results

Decide and plan
Unstable/unsure   Stable

Diagnosis required
Specific investigations

Daily management plan

Definitive treatment
Medical | Surgical | Radiological

Investigations
Blood | X-ray

Specialist opinion

Nutrition
Requirement | Route

Fluid balance prescription

Oral intake

Drugs and analgesia
Treat condition | Prophylaxis | Comorbid disease

Physiotherapy
Chest | Mobility

Drains and tubes removal

Move to a lower level of care

The CCrISP course

The CCrISP course, together with its participant handbook and other learning materials, aims to provide instruction in the practical management of critically ill and potentially ill surgical patients. CCrISP provides participants with a common-sense, consensual and safe approach to surgical critical care. The course emphasises a systematic approach to the assessment and management of patients and their problems rather than providing detailed knowledge of individual surgical conditions. Although cases may be based in one particular branch of surgery, the learning objectives are generic and relevant to all trainee surgeons. In conjunction with clinical expertise and attention to clinical detail, it is anticipated that this will help the trainee to identify patients at risk of deterioration and to prevent the development of serious complications and multiple organ failure. When patients do deteriorate, the course should help trainee surgeons to provide appropriate supportive therapy while determining the underlying cause of the deterioration and its timely management. The course advocates the involvement of senior and multidisciplinary help, at an early stage in management, to ensure that patient care is escalated appropriately and promptly. It also stresses the importance of the individual surgeon accepting responsibility for the coordination and management of the patient's care until that responsibility is formally passed to another identified individual, eg an intensive care doctor.

The participants

The course is targeted at surgical trainees from all disciplines who are in core training or equivalent staff grade posts. The course also helps surgeons prepare for higher specialty training, when they will quickly have to cope with increased clinical responsibility and decision-making. The course is designed for 16 participants and, if desired, up to 8 nurse observers. The participants are expected to read the participant handbook before the course and are required to complete a pre-course test. This ensures that they come to the course with a base level of knowledge and are therefore best placed to use the face-to-face components of the course to develop their understanding.

CCrISP instructors

CCrISP course instructors should have an interest in one or more aspects of surgical critical care and be prepared to support the course ethos. Most instructors come from a background of surgery, anaesthesia or intensive care medicine and will have regularly come into clinical contact with critically ill patients. Instructors should be at consultant level, trainees at ST5 (year 5 specialist trainee) level and above, or equivalent SAS posts, so that they have the experience to teach this course.

Teaching CCrISP provides an opportunity to motivate trainees from your own hospital or region and to reinforce the importance of high-quality continuing care for the patient at risk.

Potential instructors should preferably observe a CCrISP course and attend the CCrISP Instructor course, which has been designed to prepare instructors for the challenges of teaching CCrISP.

Some potential instructors may already have extensive experience of training and hold a qualification in education or teaching skills. Such instructors may observe a CCrISP course and then teach on a subsequent course under the supervision of the Course Director, who may then sign them off as suitable.

The course works well because of its ratio of students to teachers, interactive teaching methods and immediate clinical relevance. This maintains the participants' interest and enthusiasm and makes teaching it fun and worthwhile. The course teaching materials have been designed such that can they be taught by most faculty members and to keep the need for specialist faculty to a minimum. During your involvement with the course you will have the opportunity to teach topics that are not your first area of expertise.

All sections of the course provide the opportunity to reinforce the basic principles of surgical critical care, and this reinforcement process is actively encouraged.

Policy and procedures

The CCrISP course has set policies which your course centre, director and administrator will be familiar with. Here are a few key points.

Faculty

Directors/co-directors

The course director need not be a surgeon but, in this case, a surgeon should be identified as a co-director. The course director should have prior experience of co-directing the course and significant experience of teaching the course.

The RCS has information on the relevant roles and responsibilities of a course director.

Faculty

At least four of the faculty should have an anaesthetic/intensive care background and at least four faculty members should be surgeons. Faculty members should not receive payment for their teaching time but will be reimbursed for their travel and subsistence costs. Discretionary or professional leave (with pay but without expenses) is appropriate for teaching on this course – this is different from study leave. The RCS can provide certificates of teaching involvement and participant feedback to assist with revalidation. There are also descriptors of the roles and responsibilities of faculty members to assist with revalidation.

Consistency and standards

It is very important that this course is taught and tested in a reproducible fashion and to a common standard, as this will ensure that there is consistency in training for surgical trainees wherever they study the course. Instructors must accept that more is gained by teaching a common accepted method than by each teaching their own personal method or practice if this differs significantly from the course. All experienced doctors have their own clinical preferences, but it is best for the participants if these do not intrude inappropriately. The course is revised periodically and all instructors have the opportunity to contribute to that revision.

Copyright

All course materials are copyright of The Royal College of Surgeons of England and may not be reproduced without the prior permission of the College in writing. It is reasonable to use individual slides or the CCrISP system of assessment for appropriate teaching but the origin of the material should always be acknowledged. There is a need to maintain confidentiality of the scenario content of the courses, particularly the testing scenarios. These require an enormous amount of preparatory work to develop and pilot and confidentiality should be preserved so that they do not become common knowledge. Please do not use the scenarios for any other purpose, although if you wish to receive advice on how to build your own scenarios from your own cases then please contact the critical care tutor at the RCS, who will be happy to help.

Online support

The RCS virtual learning environment has a site dedicated to CCrISP faculty and admin. As CCrISP faculty you have authorisation to access this.

This manual contains information on the assessed parts of the course and should not be left lying around for students to see.

Teaching the CCrISP course

The aims of the CCrISP teaching materials are twofold:

1. to help ensure participants have the same learning experience wherever the course is held;
2. to help instructors prepare as quickly and as effectively as possible and, by providing the content, to allow them to focus on style of delivery.

Most participants come to the CCrISP course with rather more theoretical knowledge than practical experience. It is our job to improve their confidence and encourage them to use their knowledge in a logical way when they come across unfamiliar situations. Participants report that they find the CCrISP system of assessment extremely useful. It helps them make a logical and safe start to almost any clinical situation and allows them to bring their knowledge to bear on the problem before them. Hence the CCrISP system of assessment has a central place in the course and frequent cross-referencing to it helps the participants.

Before the course, make sure you know which lectures and small group sessions you are teaching and familiarise yourself with the relevant sections of the faculty handbook. Ensure that you check the session objectives, duration and materials required.

Using the teaching material supplied (Microsoft PowerPoint presentations, case scenarios, etc.) allows you to concentrate more on your style of delivery. In general, participants like interactive, clinically based sessions. Achieving this within the allotted time takes preparation and practice but it will be greatly appreciated by the participants.

Each session has designated objectives. It is essential that these are covered and that participants know what they are so they can focus on them.

Making a session interactive usually makes it memorable and fun. Posing appropriate questions takes a bit of practice but it is well worth the effort.

Similarly, the shift to clinical decision-making (rather than data gathering) is a key step up between junior and senior trainees. Encourage the participants to make decisions and keep the situations as realistic as possible.

No matter how good the teacher, participants usually remember a relatively modest amount of the content. Consequently, reinforcing key points at the close of the session is vital and a common error is to drop this when time is short. Always plan your closure, leave time for questions, and then give your closing points using the PowerPoint summary slide if applicable. Do not finish with questions, as the participants may leave thinking about some tangential question rather than the key points of the session.

Away from the course, participants have to satisfy numerous senior colleagues and examiners at work and in examinations. Consequently, they need accepted middle-ground approaches that they can use under a range of circumstances. The course material provides this. Participants are probably less selective than seniors about information that they discard. For these reasons it is essential that teaching follows the content of the participant and faculty handbooks. All CCrISP faculty are experienced clinicians and we have to put our personal preferences aside in order to give the participants the advantage of a unified message.

No course will be successful unless the participants value the experience. Nothing will destroy this more quickly than a bad role model, for instance faculty members who purport to teach a certain skill in a particular way but make it quite clear that they do not believe in what they are doing. The course provides one safe way of doing things – it does not state that this is the only method but simply that it has been agreed upon for this purpose.

Using teaching materials prepared by someone else is challenging. The faculty teaching notes in this document are intended to help you understand the author's intentions. Consideration of some basic principles may help you deliver the course:

- Keep scenarios as realistic as possible by trying to imagine them in real life. This is particularly challenging as the course is presented in sessions aligned to specific diagnoses and the 'feel' of a case is difficult to experience without the physical presence of the patient. Realism is particularly important in the simulated patient teaching aspects of the course and during the final assessment.

- Allow the candidates to do all the evaluation of data and clinical information. It is very easy, especially when trying to get through a lot of material, to do the analysis for the candidates and then ask them what they would do. Often it is working out what is wrong that is difficult for trainees; once they know the diagnosis, they know the treatment.

- Do not underestimate the importance of peer-to-peer learning. Significant learning takes place when candidates discuss things amongst themselves with the faculty member acting as a facilitator of the discussion.

- Use the workshops to explore candidates' understanding. Be mindful of the concept of levels of knowledge and try to explore whether candidates just know a fact or can use that knowledge appropriately and whether or not they can evaluate how useful the knowledge is.

Feedback

The overall aim of the course is to help every participant improve and to get as many as possible to complete it successfully – the course has been designed with the expectation that the great majority of participants will do so. Faculty can facilitate this by providing appropriate and timely feedback on participants' performance. When doing this you should ask the performer, and then the other participants, what went well and then ask for suggestions for improvement. You should sum up the discussion with appropriate praise and provide a maximum of three points for improvement.

It is important to listen carefully while the participant states what he or she did well. This may be one of the first indications that the participant lacks insight into their weaknesses. If the question is not asked, you will never know. It is also important to ask for points for improvement rather than 'what went badly?'. It is very easy to give a list of negative points, but this should be a time for reflection and there are important lessons to be learnt by thinking positively about ways to improve. A good question to ask is 'what would you do differently next time?'.

Case scenarios

Many elements of the course use case scenarios; these function at several levels. They make the course interesting and give clinical relevance as they have been chosen from a wide spectrum of surgical patients and they are also selected for their content. A scenario may illustrate a particular complication, pitfall or chain of events that is not necessarily part of that teaching session. Faculty need to be familiar with the scenarios they use and this can require quite a bit of preparation time. Not every scenario has been written with every last bit of clinical information but there is enough to deliver the session. Occasionally, you will need to be ready to provide further appropriate information that helps the emerging clinical picture go in the direction intended. This can be challenging as the intention is to avoid candidates jumping to conclusions and guessing what the point of the particular case presentation is. Careful use of terminology is required so preparation and familiarity with the teaching material is essential.

Using someone else's scenarios can be difficult if you do not quite 'tune in' to the author's way of thinking. If this happens, ask the course director or another faculty member they would approach it. It can be tempting to modify the scenarios provided or make up your own scenarios for the course, but this is discouraged: CCrISP scenarios have been rehearsed extensively so that areas of confusion are minimised. Most are based on real cases and the clinical, physiological and biochemical data are used faithfully.

Small group sessions

All teaching sessions should be structured and this depends on preparation. The most widely used structure is the introduction–body–summary model. During the introduction, the instructor outlines what will be covered during the session and the way in which this will relate both to clinical practice and to other parts of the course. It can also indicate the manner in which questions will be handled.

Linkage between sections helps the participant see the relevance of common themes. Your final summary should emphasise the key points covered during the session. There are usually specific summary slides in the session and a summary section should always be preceded by giving participants the opportunity to ask questions.

Small group sessions require preparation, both of content to be taught and also of the location, teaching materials and necessary props such as a laptop or other items of equipment. This is your responsibility, as is helping to store it away at the end.

The small group sessions are best run as highly interactive tutorials. The more interactive any teaching session is, the more proficient the instructor has to be to maintain control and to ensure that all of the key points are covered. Forethought and planning are essential and time the limiting factor.

At the end of the session, the instructor should sum up what has been done and the way in which it relates to the learning outcomes for the session.

Key points

- Prepare thoroughly.

- Check your materials and the environment.

- Check you have your mark sheet, where applicable.

- Keep an eye on time.

- Cross-reference to the CCrISP system of assessment, other parts of the course and to clinical practice.

- Make it interactive.

- Use of questioning – 'what are the important points here and what do you make of them...?'

- Decision-making – 'what would you do now?'

- Involve observers appropriately.

- Tidy up at the end of the session.

Assessment and certification

Participants on the course are assessed and, if they successfully complete all elements of the course, are issued with a certificate. This certificate is issued by The Royal College of Surgeons of England. Students should be encouraged to complete the online course feedback quickly to speed up the certification process.

The principal aim of the course is to make every participant a better practitioner of surgical critical care, whatever their starting point. It is important that the assessment of participants is carried out fairly and those whose performance is unsatisfactory do not complete the course.

To complete the course satisfactorily the participants must:

- attend the entire course;

- demonstrate adequate knowledge of the principles of surgical critical care;

- demonstrate the ability to manage a simulated critically ill surgical patient adequately.

Participants are assessed in a number of ways:

- Throughout the course there is continual subjective assessment of core knowledge, clinical insight and enthusiasm.

- During the small group sessions participants are graded on their core knowledge, clinical insight and enthusiasm.

- Finally, participants are assessed on their ability to use what they have learnt to assess a simulated critically ill surgical patient during the practical management patient scenarios on the final day.

Assessment is conducted by all faculty members and is discussed at faculty meetings. In practice, many participants do well. The course director must ensure that faculty are aware of the CCrISP system of assessment and the way in which it is applied throughout the course. It is important that the testing is conducted using the criterion references testing sheets to enable candidates to receive feedback. It is common for candidates who do not pass the course to ask for very detailed feedback on their performance, and it can be difficult for the course director or the RCS to defend a decision not to allow a candidate to pass the course if the testing has not been performed to a suitable standard and with a clear indication of the areas where candidate performance was unsatisfactory.

Faculty meetings and mentoring

There are faculty meetings at the start and the end of the course. It is important that you attend these meetings. Faculty also meet at the end of day one to evaluate the participants, to review the day's proceedings and to plan the next day.

You may have participants to mentor during the course. Make a point of introducing yourself at the beginning of the course and talking to participants during refreshment breaks. It is your responsibility to anticipate or identify any problems or concerns that participants may have and give appropriate advice. After the course you must give feedback to one or two participants and, possibly, those on whom you have conducted the simulated patient assessments in the final session.

The performance of participants should be continuously reviewed during the course and, where possible, remedial teaching should be given, eg at the end of the day or during meal breaks.

Final-day simulated patient scenarios

Performance in the final-day scenarios is usually the most rigorous test – it is very unusual for a participant to show unsatisfactory performance during earlier sessions and then shine in the final-day scenarios. Owing to the clinical orientation of the course, most emphasis tends to be placed on performance in the final-day scenarios.

Failure to perform an adequate simulated assessment must be discussed at the faculty meeting and the following points taken into consideration:

- Those whose performance throughout the course is poor must re-sit the course if they wish to achieve certification.

- A participant who performs in an unsatisfactory but not unsafe manner in the final simulated patient scenarios but who has performed reasonably well otherwise may be deemed successful on the strength of the rest of their performance. Provided a majority of instructors support the participant, a good performance throughout the course can salvage a relatively weak patient assessment. Clear evidence of nervousness or difficulty with role play in the final simulated patient scenarios may aid this decision but there should be no evidence to suggest the potential for actual patient harm. The final decision rests with the course director.

- If the majority of instructors do not support the participant, he or she may be asked to return to a future course to re-take a simulated patient scenario. The participant should be counselled about his or her performance and given the opportunity to retake the final simulated patient scenario again.

- A participant who misses a part of the course must attend that part at a future course before being certificated as successful.

Participants have 6 months to repeat any session; failure to do so will result in them having to resit the whole course.

The unsuccessful participant

Participants whose performance is substandard usually appreciate the opportunity to discuss this with faculty. They often appreciate a senior doctor taking a specific interest in their performance. As with all critiquing, the faculty member should indicate the areas in which the participant has strengths and not refer solely to weaknesses. Some participants will benefit from further training at their base hospital by their consultant, surgical tutor or intensive care staff, and it may be appropriate for the course director to suggest and/or arrange this. Some unsuccessful participants are resistant to feedback and additional help. Therefore, it is best stated in the pre-course documents that participants' performance may be fed back to their hospital, surgical tutor or to the postgraduate dean's office if this is believed to be necessary. The course director should speak to all unsuccessful participants as well as writing a letter to their surgical tutors and giving them written feedback on their performance. This can help stop disputes and prevent the participant claiming they thought they had successfully completed the course.

Unsuccessful participants may feel they have been treated unfairly, and, therefore, it is essential that inadequate performances be fully documented. This is primarily to permit accurate feedback to the participant but also to guard against a subsequent complaint of unfair assessment. Faculty should make adequate notes, particularly during the simulated patient assessment, to document the topics covered and the level of response given. The assessment mark sheets facilitate this and the course director should emphasise this to faculty.

Resits

If a candidate needs to resit the final patient assessment, this should be done within 6 months of the date of first assessment. The centre should be prepared to accommodate up to two resit candidates per course. The resits can be scheduled during the Course Summary and Demonstration Video sessions on Day Two.

Equipment list for all simulated patient scenarios

Equipment need not be sterile and can be reused on successive courses. Remove sharps.

It is suggested that four boxes are prepared, each containing:

- oxygen masks
  - reservoir masks
  - ward-type variable concentration masks
- suction tubing and Yankauer suckers
- oral Guedel-type airways – two adult sizes
- nasopharyngeal airway
- stethoscope
- chest drain, size 30 preferably

- chest drain tubing and bottle

- BP monitor: automatic – perhaps combined with pulse oximeter/ECG monitor
  (It is recommended that at least two pulse oximeters are available for the course – preferably as combined monitors with ECG and BP. One monitor should be capable of transducing invasive pressures. Four monitors (one for each station) would be ideal, but provided two are available you can use printouts to simulate monitor readings at the other two stations.)

- pulse oximeter and probe

- ECG electrodes (stickers)

- nasogastric tube

- IV fluid giving set × 2

- syringes: 2 × 10 mL and 2 × 20 mL

- arterial blood gas syringe

- blood bottles and forms

- intravenous cannulae

- 16G (grey) Venflons

- 20G (pink) Venflons

- central venous cannulae

- 500-mL bags of normal saline, 50% dextrose (make half up as 'blood' with food colouring or similar)

- bag of colloid solution

- pressure bag for rapid infusion

- wound dressing – Mepore® type, big and small

- abdominal drains – part-fill with fake blood as needed

- urinary catheters, catheter bag and urine meter type bag – fill with cold tea as needed

- epidural catheter tubing

- sticky tape

- clipboard and pen

- opaque stoma bag

- simple make-up for patient – pallor, blue, perspiration (33% glycerol in water in spray), blood

- plastic aprons

- non-sterile gloves, medium and large.

Additionally, the room should have:

- bed with pillows, blanket and sheet

- drip stand

- tables

- display board/screens between bays.

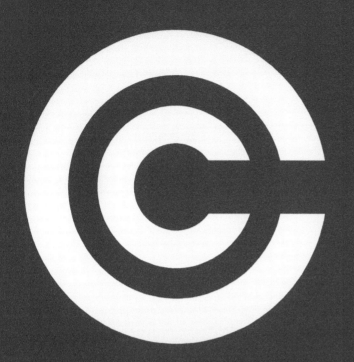

Demonstration

Introduction to CCrISP and
assessment of the critically ill
surgical patient

Introduction

This lecture is vital for establishing the premise and importance of the whole course. It should be delivered by a senior member of faculty. The scene is set by outlining the course learning outcomes and objectives but the session then moves on to a wider discussion of the importance of the CCrISP approach in delivering patient care on the wards in the modern, time-pressured hospital environment.

It is important to indicate why the course is necessary, and how this course links to early warning scores (eg the National Early Warning Score, NEWS) and the methods of responding to the deteriorating patient that the candidates are already familiar with.

During this lecture encourage interaction and reflection by the candidates, as this forms the basis for running the rest of the course. It is important to emphasise that the candidates probably already know much of what is necessary for their current stage of training and that the course is intended to develop their professionalism, clinical knowledge and non-technical skills to help prepare them for the next stage.

Duration	30 minutes
Style	Lecture
Faculty	One to deliver
AV	PowerPoint presentation

Learning outcomes

This lecture emphasises core principles of the CCrISP course. The course aims to:

- enable trainee surgeons to deal with the initial management of the acutely ill surgical patient and to predict and prevent the development of complications;

- advocate the CCrISP **three-stage assessment algorithm** for reviewing all surgical patients;

- model non-operative technical skills in a safe environment for learning.

Resources

- Laptop

- Large screen or projector

Teaching outline

The teaching material is a Microsoft PowerPoint presentation. Instructors may add their own slides if they wish to add emphasis to the learning outcomes and objectives but should not change the learning outcomes (**slides 2–4**) or summary slides.

This sets the scene that the course can help candidates cope with environments that have been created by factors such as changes in postgraduate medical training, working patterns, the demands of patients and relatives, risk management and the investigations of errors. Furthermore, the expectations of government, media and society as a whole should also be emphasised. In the UK instructors may wish to reference documents such as the **Francis Report**, the **Keogh Report** and the **Berwick Report** and the role of the **Care Quality Commission**.

Core objectives are stated as skills relevant for this stage of candidates' training, beginning with the need to identify at-risk patients, reducing the **failure to rescue** phenomenon, preventing further deterioration and minimising postoperative complications and (in some circumstances) ensuring effective end-of-life care when active treatments are deemed futile. There should also be continuing emphasis on the development of trainees' professionalism and application of holistic elements in surgical care, ie in addition to the skills and knowledge the course provides for the development of effective professional behaviours. At this juncture candidates can be made aware that, although the CCrISP course puts greater emphasis on continuity of care than other provider courses do (eg ATLS), it is not designed to turn them into intensive care medicine clinicians.

The need to rehearse patient assessment should be emphasised by reminding the candidates that most people cope badly with unfamiliar situations, and will do better if they have insight into problems and have rehearsed forms of management needed in certain situations. The course is designed to give surgical trainees a framework to deal with new (potentially life-threatening) clinical situations so that they are capable of resuscitating and stabilising patients and have the knowledge and skills to organise continuity of care, through their own efforts or the efforts of others.

This slide introduces the **CCrISP three-stage assessment algorithm**. It is worth establishing if the candidates are familiar with the algorithm already and if they routinely use it as part of their surgical practice. Lecturers may wish to emphasise its importance by informing the candidates that they themselves often apply the CCrISP three-stage assessment model in their own working lives.

The consequences of both timely and late recognition of the deteriorating adult patient should be emphasised with the physiological derangement slope, and the need to physically and mentally rehearse/visualise the approach to such circumstances should be stressed.

Slide 9

This emphasises that the CCrISP assessment system can help prevent unnoticed deterioration.

During the course it is important to remind participants of the three-stage assessment and its value. This is illustrated by the case in the next slides.

Slides 10–20

These slides present a case history to demonstrate the worst-case scenario of failure to rescue a previously fit patient. The scenario is based on a series of real events that occurred at the time of several shift changeovers (doctors, nurses and ambulance personnel) and is linked to current use of the **National Early Warning Score** (NEWS), a system not universally in place at the time of the incident. After each stage of the scenario candidates are shown a slide of a NEWS at the time of each patient review. The final score is followed by a **NEWS Escalation Plan** demonstrating that under the NEWS system the patient would have received continuous monitoring and undergone senior review, which could have been life-saving.

The slide set reinforces the worst-case consequences of failure to rescue a patient and the downward trend of deterioration, ie the longer signs of deterioration are ignored, the worse the outcome for any individual patient. The worst-case scenario of cardiac arrest (**slide 18**) should be stressed, as should the nature of the cardiac arrest, which is likely to be either asystole or pulseless electrical activity (PEA), the outcomes of which are worse than those of ventricular fibrillation or pulseless ventricular tachycardia.

National Early Warning Score	Minimum frequency of monitoring	Clinical response
0	12-hourly observations	Continue routine NEWS monitoring with every set of observations
Total: 1–4	4-hourly observations	Inform registered nurse, who must assess the patient
		Registered nurse to decide if increased frequency of monitoring and/or escalation of critical care is required
Total: 5 or more or 3 in one parameter	1-hourly observations	NEWS responder
		Response time 30 minutes
Total: 7 or more or 3 in two parameters	Continuous observations	Senior NEWS responder **and** outreach
		Response time 10 minutes

Stop! Think! Why has my patient triggered?

Slide 19

There is an opportunity at this stage to refer back to earlier slides and emphasise that this poor outcome was preventable.

Slides 20 and 21

The three-stage assessment is again shown and instructors (if time permits) could take time to ask the candidates to briefly provide examples of substandard practice from their own careers when attempts were made to 'cut corners' or a comprehensive system of assessment such as CCrISP was not used. It is recommended that this is done in pairs and the instructor invites two or three pairs to discuss their experiences. This approach should minimise the likelihood of the more vocal candidate dominating discussions if the question is asked to the entire group. Many of the case scenarios that candidates raise are likely to have a component of limited/poor communication, a problem (and solution) that can be re-emphasised during the lecture.

Slides 22 and 23

During the lecture, an overview of how to deal with the stable patient using the three-stage assessment process is also provided. Although much of the course deals with the management of the acutely ill, many trainees can suffer a relative 'paralysis of decision-making' when dealing with stable patients and the CCrISP system of assessment can help them with that.

The lecture ends with the opportunity for questions and a summary.

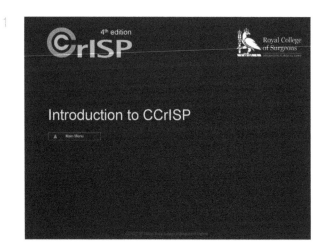

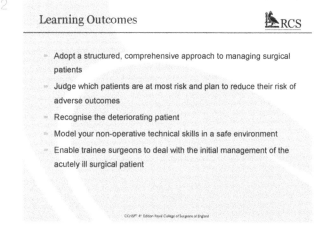

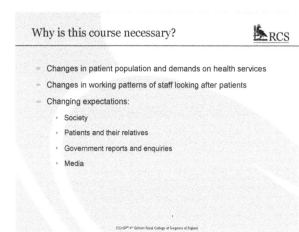

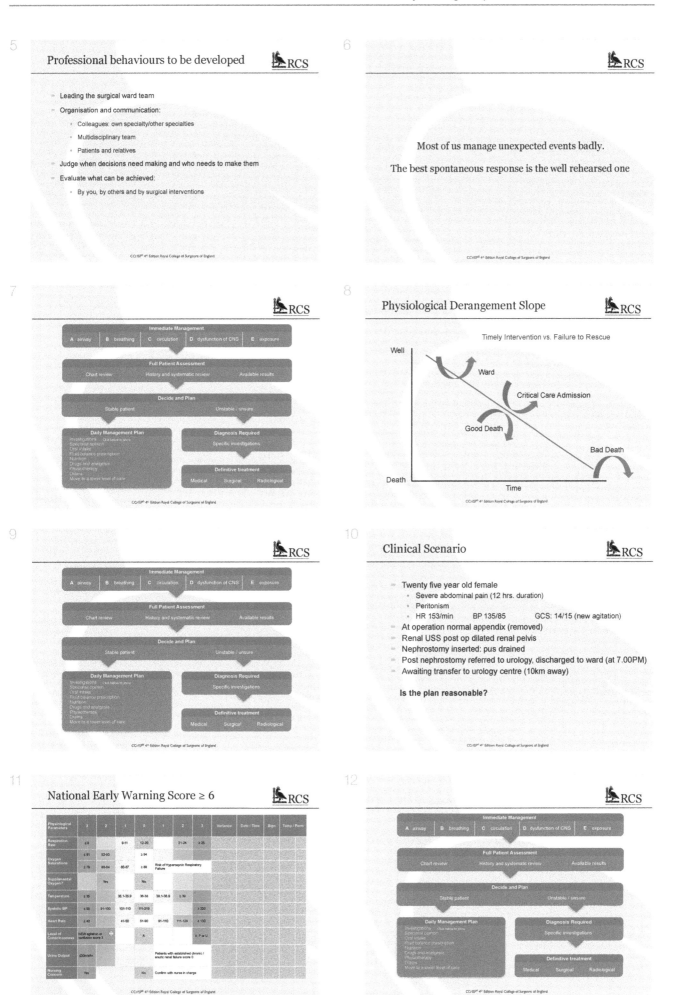

5

Professional behaviours to be developed ⬥RCS

- Leading the surgical ward team
- Organisation and communication:
  - Colleagues: own specialty/other specialties
  - Multidisciplinary team
  - Patients and relatives
- Judge when decisions need making and who needs to make them
- Evaluate what can be achieved:
  - By you, by others and by surgical interventions

6

⬥RCS

Most of us manage unexpected events badly.

The best spontaneous response is the well rehearsed one

7

⬥RCS

| Immediate Management |
| A airway | B breathing | C circulation | D dysfunction of CNS | E exposure |

| Full Patient Assessment |
| Chart review | History and systematic review | Available results |

| Decide and Plan |
| Stable patient | Unstable / unsure |

| Daily Management Plan | Diagnosis Required |
| | Specific investigations |

| Definitive treatment |
| Medical | Surgical | Radiological |

8

Physiological Derangement Slope ⬥RCS

Timely Intervention vs. Failure to Rescue

Well — Ward — Critical Care Admission — Good Death — Bad Death — Death — Time

9

⬥RCS

| Immediate Management |
| A airway | B breathing | C circulation | D dysfunction of CNS | E exposure |

| Full Patient Assessment |
| Chart review | History and systematic review | Available results |

| Decide and Plan |
| Stable patient | Unstable / unsure |

| Daily Management Plan | Diagnosis Required |
| | Specific investigations |

| Definitive treatment |
| Medical | Surgical | Radiological |

10

Clinical Scenario ⬥RCS

- Twenty five year old female
  - Severe abdominal pain (12 hrs. duration)
  - Peritonism
  - HR 153/min   BP 135/85   GCS: 14/15 (new agitation)
- At operation normal appendix (removed)
- Renal USS post op dilated renal pelvis
- Nephrostomy inserted: pus drained
- Post nephrostomy referred to urology, discharged to ward (at 7.00PM)
- Awaiting transfer to urology centre (10km away)

Is the plan reasonable?

11

National Early Warning Score ≥ 6 ⬥RCS

12

⬥RCS

| Immediate Management |
| A airway | B breathing | C circulation | D dysfunction of CNS | E exposure |

| Full Patient Assessment |
| Chart review | History and systematic review | Available results |

| Decide and Plan |
| Stable patient | Unstable / unsure |

| Daily Management Plan | Diagnosis Required |
| | Specific investigations |

| Definitive treatment |
| Medical | Surgical | Radiological |

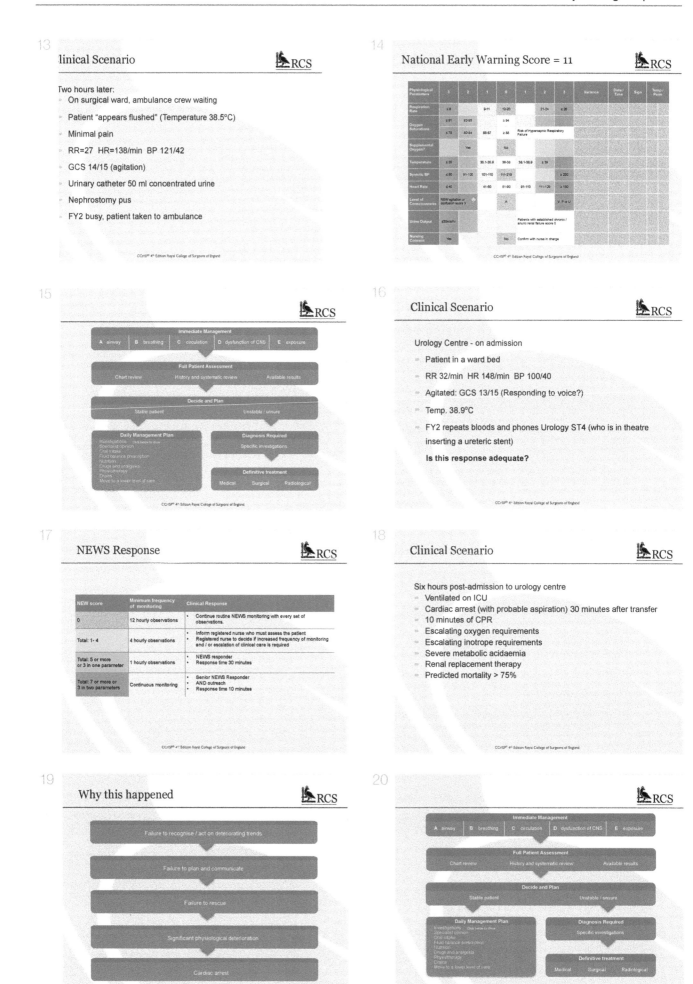

13

linical Scenario

Two hours later:
- On surgical ward, ambulance crew waiting
- Patient "appears flushed" (Temperature 38.5°C)
- Minimal pain
- RR=27 HR=138/min BP 121/42
- GCS 14/15 (agitation)
- Urinary catheter 50 ml concentrated urine
- Nephrostomy pus
- FY2 busy, patient taken to ambulance

14

National Early Warning Score = 11

15

Immediate Management

| A airway | B breathing | C circulation | D dysfunction of CNS | E exposure |

Full Patient Assessment

| Chart review | History and systematic review | Available results |

Decide and Plan

| Stable patient | Unstable / unsure |

Daily Management Plan
- Investigations
- Specialist opinion
- Oral intake
- Fluid balance prescription
- Nutrition
- Drugs and analgesia
- Physiotherapy
- Drains
- Move to a lower level of care

Diagnosis Required
- Specific investigations

Definitive treatment

| Medical | Surgical | Radiological |

16

Clinical Scenario

Urology Centre - on admission
- Patient in a ward bed
- RR 32/min HR 148/min BP 100/40
- Agitated: GCS 13/15 (Responding to voice?)
- Temp. 38.9°C
- FY2 repeats bloods and phones Urology ST4 (who is in theatre inserting a ureteric stent)
- **Is this response adequate?**

17

NEWS Response

NEW score	Minimum frequency of monitoring	Clinical Response
0	12 hourly observations	• Continue routine NEWS monitoring with every set of observations.
Total: 1- 4	4 hourly observations	• Inform registered nurse who must assess the patient • Registered nurse to decide if increased frequency of monitoring and / or escalation of clinical care is required
Total: 5 or more or 3 in one parameter	1 hourly observations	• NEWS responder • Response time 30 minutes
Total: 7 or more or 3 in two parameters	Continuous monitoring	• Senior NEWS Responder • AND outreach • Response time 10 minutes

18

Clinical Scenario

Six hours post-admission to urology centre
- Ventilated on ICU
- Cardiac arrest (with probable aspiration) 30 minutes after transfer
- 10 minutes of CPR
- Escalating oxygen requirements
- Escalating inotrope requirements
- Severe metabolic acidaemia
- Renal replacement therapy
- Predicted mortality > 75%

19

Why this happened

- Failure to recognise / act on deteriorating trends
- Failure to plan and communicate
- Failure to rescue
- Significant physiological deterioration
- Cardiac arrest

20

Immediate Management

| A airway | B breathing | C circulation | D dysfunction of CNS | E exposure |

Full Patient Assessment

| Chart review | History and systematic review | Available results |

Decide and Plan

| Stable patient | Unstable / unsure |

Daily Management Plan
- Investigations
- Specialist opinion
- Oral intake
- Fluid balance prescription
- Nutrition
- Drugs and analgesia
- Physiotherapy
- Drains
- Move to a lower level of care

Diagnosis Required
- Specific investigations

Definitive treatment

| Medical | Surgical | Radiological |

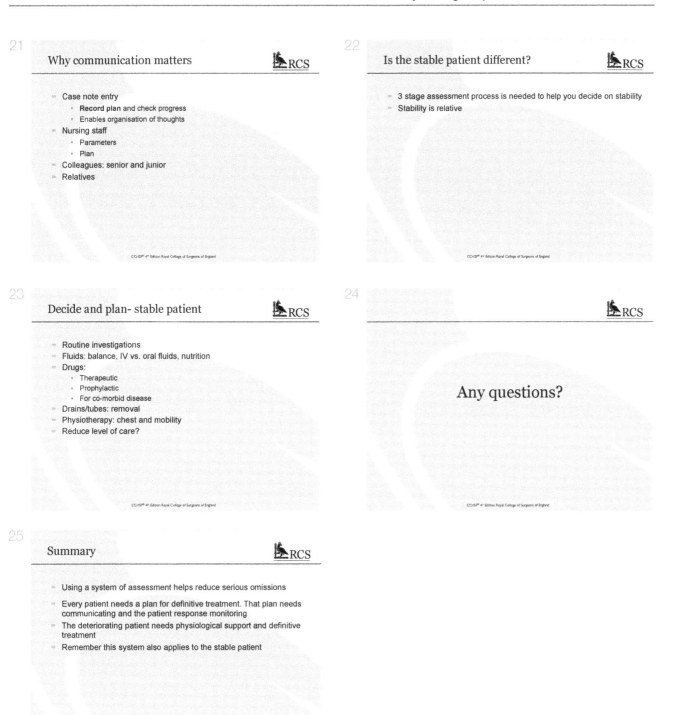

21

Why communication matters RCS

- Case note entry
  - **Record plan** and check progress
  - Enables organisation of thoughts
- Nursing staff
  - Parameters
  - Plan
- Colleagues: senior and junior
- Relatives

CCrISP® 4ᵗʰ Edition Royal College of Surgeons of England

22

Is the stable patient different? RCS

- 3 stage assessment process is needed to help you decide on stability
- Stability is relative

CCrISP® 4ᵗʰ Edition Royal College of Surgeons of England

23

Decide and plan- stable patient RCS

- Routine investigations
- Fluids: balance, IV vs. oral fluids, nutrition
- Drugs:
  - Therapeutic
  - Prophylactic
  - For co-morbid disease
- Drains/tubes: removal
- Physiotherapy: chest and mobility
- Reduce level of care?

CCrISP® 4ᵗʰ Edition Royal College of Surgeons of England

24

RCS

Any questions?

CCrISP® 4ᵗʰ Edition Royal College of Surgeons of England

25

Summary RCS

- Using a system of assessment helps reduce serious omissions
- Every patient needs a plan for definitive treatment. That plan needs communicating and the patient response monitoring
- The deteriorating patient needs physiological support and definitive treatment
- Remember this system also applies to the stable patient

CCrISP® 4ᵗʰ Edition Royal College of Surgeons of England

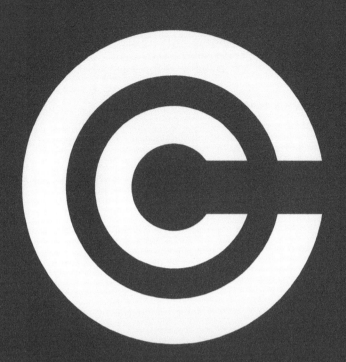

1.2

Faculty demonstration
Patient assessment

Introduction

In this part of the session, the faculty demonstrate the CCrISP system of assessment on a simulated patient. After this participants are split into four groups of four, and each participant will have an opportunity to conduct a supervised (and assisted) assessment of a patient who requires immediate resuscitation and in whom the underlying cause of deterioration needs to be identified.

Duration	20 minutes
Style	Demonstration
Faculty	Three or four
	• one to introduce and conduct questions
	• one participant
	• one nurse
	• one patient (if patient models are used, then only three members of faculty are needed)
AV	None

Learning outcomes

▪ To demonstrate the recommended CCrISP system of assessment on a simulated patient.

▪ To emphasise key concepts discussed in the preceding lecture.

▪ To demonstrate and stress the importance of role play during the course.

▪ To introduce the principles of feedback.

Teaching outline

The exercise requires four people to fulfil the roles: an instructor, a doctor/participant, a patient and a nurse practitioner. The scenario is easiest to run if instructors take on these roles.

Time is limited so the faculty involved in this part of the course need to prepare and rehearse just before the course starts or during the preceding lecture.

One instructor should give a short introduction, indicating the aims and relating this exercise to the lecture just given and the practical session that follows. The instructor should indicate that they will be looking for comments from the participants on the demonstration.

Then allow the scenario to run: the doctor/participant is given information by the nurse and then assesses/manages the patient using the CCrISP system. As time is short it is best if the nurse relays findings and controls the tempo as needed. The patient should have rehearsed one or two simple cues for tachypnoea, rigors, etc, as the scenario dictates.

Stop the scenario at a point which allows enough time for discussion of the system and of the specifics of the case, including ABCs, underlying cause and making a plan of action. Involve as many participants as you can. It is useful if you get beyond the ABCs and into full assessment as there are a number of points to be made. In particular, the narcotisation does not explain the hypovolaemia and this needs to be assessed, a cause diagnosed, and then managed.

Leave time to take a few questions and then summarise the objectives at the end. Possible topics for the concluding comments are shown in the brief. It is always helpful to emphasise that use of a system helps avoid simple errors and that underlying causes of deterioration must be found and dealt with.

Timeline

Introduction	3 minutes
Scenario	10 minutes
Discussion	5 minutes
Questions and closure	2 minutes

Resources

▶ CCrISP system of assessment poster.

▶ Equipment list as per the assessment scenarios and the following notes.

▶ Demonstration scenario documents:

- 1.2.0 History sheet.

- 1.2.1 Prescription chart.

- 1.2.2 Fluid chart.

- 1.2.3 Observation chart.

Demonstration scenario: narcotisation with hypovolaemia (slow drip + possible bleeding ulcer)

Patient brief

You had a hip replacement yesterday and have had a lot of pain. You are now unconscious with very slow breathing because of a morphine overdose. When you wake up in response to treatment you still feel very unwell with abdominal pain in the upper part of the abdomen. If asked, this abdominal pain has been there for about 12 hours.

Make-up

- Small IV cannula left hand.
- Patient blue and sweaty.
- Wound drain in left hip.
- Urinary catheter.

Documents available

▶ 1.2.0 History sheet.

▶ 1.2.1 Prescription chart.

▶ 1.2.2 Fluid chart.

▶ 1.2.3 Observation chart.

Background for instructor

The patient has increasing pain due to a poorly running drip and patient-controlled analgesia (PCA). A bolus of morphine causes a respiratory periarrest.

Appropriate immediate management of this respiratory problem (naloxone) reveals a secondary issue: worsening hypotension and rising heart rate due to:

- dehydration due to a slow-running IV drip;

- a possible peptic ulcer bleed secondary to NSAID administration (in retrospect worsening pain may have been abdominal in origin).

Cardiac pain is also a possibility.

Brief for the participant

You are the orthopaedic junior registrar and have been summoned to the bed of a patient who has had a recent routine left hip replacement. The patient has just been found poorly responsive on the ward. Analgesia has been difficult and the morphine PCA was not controlling the pain and the patient needed an additional bolus. The nurse informs you that the drip has not been running well.

Immediate management

A Airway is inadequate. Airway manoeuvres are required to improve the situation. No foreign bodies or liquids can be seen in the mouth. A Guedel may be inserted but will be spat out after naloxone is given.

B High-flow oxygen to be administered. Respiratory rate 5/min. Chest examination shows equal air entry but shallow breathing. Oxygen saturation is initially 90% on air and 99% on 15 litres of inspired oxygen.

Participants should recognise that the patient has an upper airway problem and should initiate treatment promptly:

C Underperfused. Peripherally shut down with heart rate 115/min regular. BP 90/60. Patient feels cool with capillary return of 4 seconds. Intravenous fluid challenge should be initiated. Legs can be raised (in ALS guidelines). Parameters improve with fluid to HR 100/min and BP 105/70.

D Pupils constricted. U on AVPU. Responds rapidly to naloxone in titrated doses (50–100 µg IV). When awake will complain of pain in epigastrium.

E In pyjamas with left hip wound and drain (drain has old blood <400 mL).

Definitive assessment

1.2.0 History sheet. This shows the admission clerking by a foundation doctor with allergies marked as penicillin and Septrin. Patient has osteoarthritis and has just undergone a routine left hip replacement. The patient has a history of peptic ulcer disease and until recently was taking omeprazole (a proton pump inhibitor). This was stopped by the patient's GP 2 weeks ago. Other meds: lisinopril and paracetamol.

1.2.1 Prescription chart. Recent diclofenac given. Morphine bolus given in past 30 minutes. On morphine PCA.

1.2.2 Fluid chart. Slow-running fluids.

1.2.3 Observation chart. Dropping respiratory rate and saturations. Recent-onset hypotension. Increasing heart rate. Increasing NEWS (early warning score).

Discuss

▣ Management of the airway emergency (and opiate overdose).

▣ Treatment of hypotension.

▣ Causes of hypotension in this patient (dehydration, peptic ulceration secondary to NSAIDs, exclude cardiac causes).

This scenario is to be run as a demonstration of the three-part CCrISP assessment algorithm and it may be useful to stop the scenario after each part of the assessment to involve the audience in the management of the patient.

Emphasise the use of CCrISP to assess and treat the patient in a systematic manner.

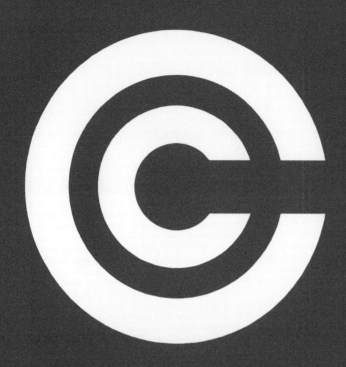

Initial patient scenarios
Assessment of the critically ill surgical patient – practical management

Introduction

In this session, the participants should be divided into four groups of four. Each candidate will have an opportunity to conduct a supervised (and assisted) assessment of a patient who requires immediate resuscitation and in whom the underlying factor needs to be identified.

Duration	80 minutes (four 20-minute rotations)
Style	Practical (participants do the patient assessment and management)
Faculty	Eight in total:
	• minimum of two per group
	• one faculty member as scenario manager
	• one faculty member or model as patient
AV	NA

Learning outcomes

- To emphasise key concepts discussed in the lecture on patient assessment, in particular simultaneous assessment and immediate management with a search for an underlying cause.

- To introduce some of the topics that will be covered during the rest of the course.

Teaching outline

Each group rotates around four scenarios and in each scenario a different member of the group takes on the role of assessing the patient. In this way, every candidate has an opportunity to manage a critically ill patient using the CCrISP system of assessment. The other group members should be encouraged to comment constructively on the assessed candidate's performance.

The scenarios consist of four straightforward cases which have been written to demonstrate a problem in airway, breathing, circulation or dysfunction. Each scenario contains an important abnormality, detectable and correctable during immediate management, and simple notes or chart review.

One instructor teaches/runs the scenario while another person (usually the second instructor) plays the patient. Centres may use medical students or other staff to simulate the patient. The first instructor should relay information as the participant examines the patient in as near to 'real time' as possible. The instructor must also keep time as it is easy to overrun during this session. Numbers permitting, a third person may play the role of a nurse (in some centres nurse observers are asked to play this role).

Preparation

Instructors must review and rehearse their scenario beforehand and prepare the session during the initial lecture. This is probably the most time-pressured and difficult part of the course to get right, so **preparation is essential**. Keep the first run-through of the scenario simple: the participants will be slower during the first scenario while they get used to what is expected of them. Some participants will need to be guided through while others will have a very hands-off approach and try to conduct a 'viva over the patient'. Many will need help with the steps of the CCrISP system of assessment and you should have the CCrISP poster above the bed. Candidates often stick at the immediate management phase – not wanting to progress until the ABCs are normalised – encourage them to act normally and get on and begin a definitive assessment while they see what the effects of their initial manoeuvres are, assuming this is safe.

Details of the scenarios are given below.

At the start

The instructor should briefly set out the aims of the whole session. The main objective of this session and at this stage of the course is to help the candidates to assess a patient systematically and gather the relevant information accurately so that they can build it into a simple and logical plan.

At the end

At the end of each scenario, the instructor should recap some of the general aims covered in the scenario as well as the specific learning points. Between rotations, review whether the scenario is getting across the message you want. At the end, the lead instructor at each patient scenario should sum up, indicating that the rest of the course will flesh out many of the problems touched on during this session.

Four scenarios follow: participants rotate, instructors work through the same scenario four times with a different group each time. If there are new instructors, let them watch the first two and then run the next two, with assistance if needed.

Timeline

Each 20-minute rotation consists of:

Introduction, select participant	1 minute
Brief participant	1 minute
Participant performs scenario	13 minutes
Feedback and questions	4 minutes
Summary	1 minute

Resources

▶ CCrISP system of assessment poster

Scenario A

▶ 1.3.0 History sheet.

▶ 1.3.1 Prescription chart.

Scenario B

▶ 1.4.0 History sheet.

▶ 1.4.1 Observation (NEWS) chart.

▶ 1.4.2 Results: ABGs, Hb, chest X-ray report.

▶ 1.4.3 Drug chart.

Scenario C

▶ 1.5.0 Observation chart.

▶ 1.5.1 Drug chart.

▶ 1.5.2 ERCP report.

▶ 1.5.3 Results sheet.

Scenario D

▶ 1.6.0 Clerking history.

▶ 1.6.1 Surgical operation note.

▶ 1.6.2 Postoperative history.

▶ 1.6.3 Prescription chart.

▶ 1.6.4 ABGs.

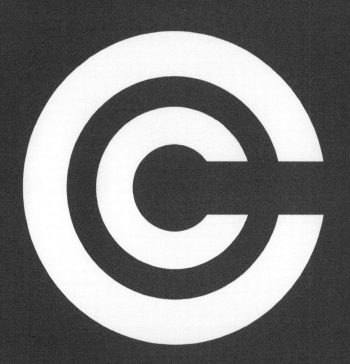

1.3

Scenario A
**Stridor secondary to anaphylaxis
to penicillin**

Patient brief

You are a patient on an orthopaedic ward readmitted 1 week after a left total hip replacement and have developed a wound infection. You have just been given an injection of a penicillin antibiotic (tazocin: piperacillin–tazobactam) and have started to struggle with your breathing.

You feel hot and distressed and are experiencing stridor (upper airway obstruction leading to problems breathing in and getting your breath). You are having an anaphylactic reaction to the antibiotic.

You are clothed, on a hospital bed and have a patent IV cannula. Once you are given oxygen, adrenaline and steroid and antihistamine injections your breathing improves. If you do not receive the appropriate treatment you will become unresponsive and eventually stop breathing.

Make-up

- IV cannula left hand.

Documents available

▶ 1.3.0 History sheet. This shows the admission clerking by a foundation doctor with allergies marked as penicillin and Septrin. An entry from later the same day shows that the orthopaedic consultant during the ward round diagnosed left hip wound infection and prescribed tazocin to be started after cultures are taken (note that although tazocin is a broad-spectrum antibiotic, and probably not indicated for a wound infection, it is put into the scenario as many medical staff do not realise it contains a penicillin).

▶ 1.3.1 Prescription chart. This shows administration of tazocin 4.5 g, which is in progress when the patient is reviewed.

Background for instructor

The patient has a wound infection following a left total hip replacement. The patient is otherwise well with no other medical problems of note. The history includes a vague mention of penicillin allergy (the admission notes say '?rash as a child') but the patient has been prescribed intravenous piperacillin–tazobactam (tazocin), and is experiencing an anaphylactic reaction to this. This initially manifests as mild respiratory distress but progresses to severe stridor if the candidate does not recognise this as a possibility.

Oxygen saturations will decrease rapidly if the condition is not promptly treated with oxygen, adrenaline, steroids and antihistamines after chart review. If treated correctly, the patient will improve.

- The scenario is designed to test the airway and breathing components of the CCrISP algorithm.

- Although the patient has anaphylaxis, the primary clinical issues are the airway and breathing. Candidates should not be allowed to become fixated on haemodynamic compromise to the detriment of correctly managing the airway and respiratory problems.

- The challenge is to recognise anaphylaxis with airway compromise rapidly and to treat this as a potentially life-threatening condition.

Brief for the participant

You are the orthopaedic junior registrar and have been summoned to the bed of a 60-year-old patient readmitted earlier in the day with a wound infection 7 days after a left total hip repair. The nurse at the bedside tells you the patient has suddenly became very short of breath and wheezy just after putting up some tazocin.

Immediate management

A   Patient has wheeze, can speak only in short sentences and keeps complaining of a tight chest. The patient's lips are swollen and face is flushed. Airway is adequate (just) but threatened. No tracheal tug. Airway manoeuvres do not help. No foreign bodies or liquids can be seen in the mouth.

B   High-flow oxygen to be administered. Respiratory rate 30/min. Chest examination shows equal air entry with severe stridor/wheeze on auscultation. Oxygen saturation is 90% on air and 95% on 15 litres of inspired oxygen. The patient does not have chest pain.

Participants should recognise that the patient has an upper airway problem and should initiate treatment promptly: at this stage of the assessment it would be reasonable to administer nebulised salbutamol or even nebulised adrenaline.

C   Heart rate 130/min regular. BP 90/35. Patient feels flushed with capillary return of 4 seconds. IV fluid challenge should be initiated. Legs can be raised (in ALS guidelines).

D   Distressed, awake but deteriorates rapidly to drowsiness and coma if condition is not treated promptly.

E   In pyjamas with left painful hip wound.

Chart review

- Drug chart with documented allergy to penicillin.

- Signed for first dose of tazocin.

Definitive assessment

- If asked, the nurse will confirm that patient has just had IV antibiotic.

- If asked, the patient will confirm allergy to penicillin and Septrin.

- Penicillin allergy is clearly marked in the notes and recent administration of tazocin should confirm the diagnosis of anaphylaxis.

- At this point candidate should mention the treatment that is needed:

  - adrenaline (0.5 mL of 1:1000 adrenaline IM)

  - hydrocortisone (200 mg IV)

  - chlorphenamine (10 mg IV)

  - further nebulised adrenaline can be administered but alone will not improve the patient's condition.

Discuss

- Management of the airway emergency.

- Use of a system of assessment to make rapid, safe assessment without jumping to conclusions.

- Importance of allergy history.

- Treatment of anaphylaxis.

- Prevention of drug errors.

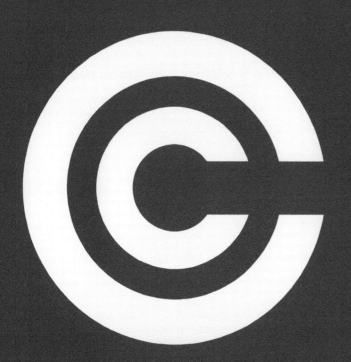

Scenario B
Haemothorax secondary to a rib fracture following a fall in a urology patient

Patient brief

You are an elderly patient admitted from a residential care home with urinary retention and a urinary tract infection secondary to benign prostatic disease. You have been catheterised.

Whilst attempting to move to a chair 2 hours earlier you slipped on the floor and fell against the bed. You were seen by a junior doctor, who prescribed paracetamol and ordered a chest X-ray.

You have fractured a right rib, which is increasingly affecting your breathing. You have a haemothorax as you are on dual antiplatelet therapy for ischaemic heart disease. You are awake, lucid and clothed on your hospital bed. You have a urinary catheter in place and a slow-running IV drip. You are very anxious.

Once you have been given pain relief the rib fracture pain improves but the shortness of breath does not improve. Definitive management once the chest X-ray report is seen should be right chest drain insertion.

Make-up

- Slight cyanosis.

Documents available

▶ 1.4.0 History sheet.

▶ 1.4.1 Observation (NEWS) chart.

▶ 1.4.2 Results: ABGs, Hb, chest X-ray report.

▶ 1.4.3 Drug chart.

Background for instructor

The patient is a 78-year-old man with prostatic urinary retention and urinary tract infection who has just been catheterised on the surgical admissions unit. He has a history of ischaemic heart disease and is on clopidogrel and aspirin. He had a fall whilst transferring to a chair 2 hours previously, injuring his right chest. He was seen by the junior doctor, who ordered a chest X-ray. The nursing staff has called for the surgical registrar as his pain is worse and he is now short of breath. The patient has developed a haemothorax secondary to a rib fracture and the pharmacological combination of clopidogrel and aspirin (in his admission history). The chest X-ray report confirms this diagnosis.

The patient is able to inform the candidate of his fall and the increasing shortness of breath.

Initial CCrISP respiratory management and examination will reveal a hypoxic patient with a dull right chest on percussion with decreased breath sound on the same side. Palpation of the chest will identify an acutely tender area in the right anterior axillary line consistent with a rib fracture.

The patient is tachycardic but otherwise haemodynamically stable.

The patient will respond to pain relief and high-flow oxygen. A chest X-ray should be ordered to confirm the diagnosis prior to referral for chest drain insertion.

Emergency needle thoracostomy for erroneously suspected pneumothorax will result in a rapid decrease in the patient's clinical status with increasing hypoxia.

Brief for the participant

You have been called to the surgical admissions ward to review a 78-year-old man with prostatic urinary retention. He has been catheterised but whilst transferring to a chair fell and hurt his right chest. He is now very short of breath and in significant pain.

Immediate management

A   Airway maintained, talking in short sentences.

B   Short of breath. SpO$_2$ 92%. High-flow oxygen to be administered, following which saturations improve to 96%. Trachea central. Dull right chest on percussion. Decreased breath sound on right on auscultation.

C   HR 120/min. Decreased peripheral perfusion with prolonged capillary return at 3 seconds. BP 110/90. A 20G (pink) IVI with Hartmann's solution is in place, running slowly. Large-bore cannulae can be easily inserted. Fluid challenge should be given, following which the heart rate decreases to 100/min and the peripheral perfusion improves.

D   Patient is anxious and in considerable pain. A on AVPU. Pupils are normal in size and normally reactive to light.

E   In pyjamas. Urinary catheter in place (clear urine). IVI.

Pulse oximetry/monitoring should be attached. Full blood profile including a cross-match and arterial blood gas should be requested.

Full patient assessment

▪   The chart review shows that the deterioration started immediately after the fall.

▪   Clerking history notes ischaemic heart disease and shows that the patient is on dual antiplatelet therapy; this is confirmed by the drug chart.

▪   Arterial blood gas shows hypoxia with a normal PaCO$_2$.

▪   Haemoglobin is 90 g/L.

▪   The chest X-ray report shows a right-sided haemothorax secondary to a rib fracture.

Decide and plan

- The candidate should recognise that the patient requires an urgent chest drain but that this should only be performed with senior assistance.

- Haematological advice may be necessary with regard to reversing the dual antiplatelet therapy.

- It should be recognised that the patient is at risk of cardiac ischaemia and an ECG should be requested.

- The patient should be referred to a higher care bed (HDU) as he is clearly unstable.

- The candidate should administer pain relief in the form of titrated morphine. Paracetamol has been prescribed but not yet given.

Discuss

- Importance of immediate management in critically ill patient.

- Recognition of the unstable patient and the need for higher care transfer.

- Complicating comorbidities in elderly surgical patients (ischaemic heart disease).

- Bleeding risk with antiplatelet therapy.

- The need to review any investigations that have been ordered (eg the chest X-ray).

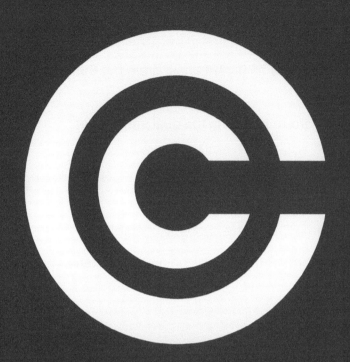

Scenario C

Sepsis in a hepatobiliary patient

Patient brief

You are a 45-year-old admitted from home under the hepatobiliary surgical service with an obstructed bile duct due to an impacted gallstone. Prior to admission you were fit and well.

Four hours earlier you underwent endoscopic retrograde cholangiopancreatography (ERCP) under sedation to treat the blockage.

You are now back on the surgical ward and are feeling very unwell. You have been vomiting and feel hot and very shivery. This is due to infection from the bile duct.

Make-up

- Sweaty.

Documents available

▶ 1.5.0 Observation chart.

▶ 1.5.1 Prescription chart.

▶ 1.5.2 ERCP report.

▶ 1.5.3 Blood results sheet.

Background for instructor

The patient is a 45-year-old patient with biliary sepsis following ERCP without appropriate antibiotic cover. The patient is acutely unwell, nauseated and is having rigors.

Examination will reveal a septic and hypotensive patient. The patient is hot and sweaty with a temperature of 38.5°C and has abdominal pain and tenderness in the right upper quadrant.

Brief for the participant

You have been called to the surgical admissions ward to review a previously well 45-year-old patient with biliary obstruction treated 4 hours earlier with ERCP. The patient was admitted the day before with a 1-week history of right upper quadrant pain. The nurse is very concerned as the patient is sweaty and looks extremely unwell.

Immediate management

A   Airway maintained, talking in sentences.

B   RR 25/min. Saturations cannot be read because of the patient's shivering. There is no cyanosis although the patient looks pale and sweaty. Thoracic examination is normal. High-flow oxygen to be administered.

C   HR 140 bpm. Decreased peripheral perfusion with prolonged capillary return at 5 seconds. BP 90/30. There is a 22G (blue) IV cannula with no intravenous solution attached. Large-bore cannulae can be easily inserted. Fluid challenge should be given, following which the heart rate decreases to 110/min, BP increases to 100/40, the peripheral perfusion improves and the patient reports feeling better.

D   Patient is anxious and feels unwell. A on AVPU. Pupils are normal in size and normally reactive to light.

E   Pyrexial at 38.5°C. No urinary catheter. Abdominal pain in right upper quadrant on palpation. If not already done, full monitoring should be attached. Full blood profile and arterial blood gas should be requested.

Full patient assessment

- The ERCP notes state that the procedure was successful with no obvious complications.

- The prescription chart shows that 2 mg of midazolam and 25 mg of fentanyl were administered during ERCP. Gentamicin 240 mg is written on the front of the chart but has not been signed for (ie was not given).

- Arterial blood gas shows good oxygenation and compensated metabolic acidosis with a lactate of 3 and a bicarbonate of 19.

- WCC is raised at 17.

- Raised ALP and a bilirubin of 25; amylase normal.

- Hb and platelets are normal.

Decide and plan

- The candidate should recognise that the patient has biliary sepsis secondary to the procedure and lack of antibiotic cover.

- After initial oxygen management and fluid resuscitation the patient improves.

- Blood cultures should be requested prior to administration of an IV antibiotic (eg gentamicin, cephalosporin, co-amoxiclav). It would be reasonable to consult microbiology or antibiotic protocol prior to this prescription.

- The patient should be catheterised.

- The patient should be discussed with the critical care team.

- The candidate should administer pain relief in the form of titrated morphine.

Discuss

- Importance of rapid diagnosis and treatment of suspected sepsis (within 1 hour).

- 'Sepsis 6' guidelines can be mentioned if there is time:

  - high-flow O_2

  - blood cultures

  - empirical antibiotics

  - serum lactate and full blood count

  - IV fluid resuscitation

  - urinary catheterisation.

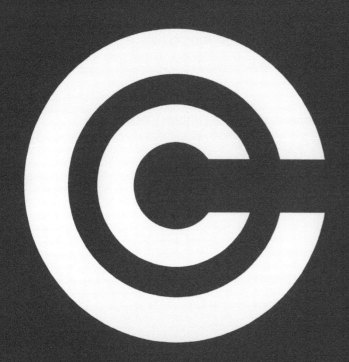

Scenario D
Narcotised patient with retained secretions

Patient brief

You have chronic bronchitis and 2 days ago had a laparotomy for an incarcerated umbilical hernia with incipient bowel obstruction. You have received too much opiate analgesia, which is affecting your breathing.

You are initially unresponsive with noisy, slow, 'see-saw' respirations. If your airway is cleared and oxygen is given you become a bit more responsive.

Make-up

- IV cannula left hand.
- Blue (cyanosed).
- Catheterised with urine bag.

Documents available

▶ 1.6.0 Clerking history. This shows that the patient has severe chronic obstructive pulmonary disease (COPD) and takes regular inhalers. Admitted with incipient bowel obstruction secondary to an incarcerated hernia.

▶ 1.6.1 Surgical operation note. Uncomplicated laparotomy for incarcerated hernia. No bowel resection or anastomosis was required. Bowel was healthy.

▶ 1.6.2 Postoperative history. Postoperative ileus, nasogastric tube pulled out by patient in sleep. Nil by mouth. Delay in PCA set-up, leading to morphine 10 mg bolus being given 2 hours prior to your review.

▶ 1.6.3 Drug kardex. The chart shows that postoperative respiratory meds have been refused. It also shows that a one-off dose of morphine 10 mg IV was given 2 hours ago.

▶ 1.6.4 ABGs. This shows a type 2 respiratory failure (hypoxia + respiratory acidosis).

Background for instructor

This patient has COPD and is close to having a respiratory arrest as a result of a decreased consciousness level (opiate narcotisation) exacerbated by lack of bronchodilators and diaphragmatic splinting due to a postoperative ileus.

The initial management should consist of high-flow oxygen and airway manoeuvres (chin lift, jaw thrust, oropharyngeal or nasopharyngeal airway insertion), following which the patient will improve slightly.

The candidate should realise that the patient is narcotised as a result of the recent IV morphine bolus and should administer titrated naloxone.

Further management includes nebulised bronchodilators, reinsertion of the nasogastric tube and referral to a high-dependency unit.

Brief for the participant

It is 1 pm. You are the general surgical registrar and are urgently called to see a 65-year-old patient with chronic bronchitis 2 days after an emergency laparotomy for an incarcerated umbilical hernia. The patient has become unresponsive on the ward. The nurse reports that the patient has been drowsy for an hour but has recently deteriorated.

The patient had previously been doing relatively well although pain and abdominal distension had been an issue. The patient had returned from theatre with an epidural, which was removed today. The acute pain team has just set up a PCA.

Immediate management

A   Patient is unresponsive with noisy breathing and an obstructed breathing pattern. On inspection there is nothing in the airway and a chin lift/jaw thrust improves the breathing pattern slightly. The patient will tolerate an oro- or nasopharyngeal airway, significantly improving breathing.

B   High-flow oxygen to be administered. Respiratory rate is 10/min. Chest examination shows equal air entry with wheeze on auscultation. Oxygen saturations are initially 70% but improve rapidly to 90% when the airway is opened. If given, nebulisers improve the wheeze.

C   Heart rate 110/min regular. BP 100/50. Capillary return of 3 seconds. Intravenous fluid challenge should be initiated following which HR and BP improve. Blood samples, arterial blood gases and chest X-ray should be requested. The blood gas shows a respiratory acidosis (the only available results).

D   Initially unresponsive on AVPU. Pupils very constricted. Airway manoeuvres improve consciousness level to P on AVPU. Administration of naloxone (100 µg boluses) results in the patient waking and responding to voice. Administration of a large (400-µg) bolus of naloxone results in severe abdominal pain over the wound.

E   Abdominal wound. Catheter in place with urine in bag. Belly sore over wound and **very** distended but not peritonitic.

Definitive assessment

The candidate should realise that this patient needs on-going care in a high-dependency area. The patient is likely to have on-going issues with pain, abdominal distension and the underlying COPD and the naloxone will eventually wear off. The patient is not stable.

Discuss

- Management of the airway emergency.

- Management of narcotisation and low consciousness level.

▢ Importance of understanding a patient's medical history and usual medications and how comorbidities affect perioperative management of surgical patients.

▢ The effect of diaphragmatic splinting (distended abdomen due to ileus) on respiratory effort.

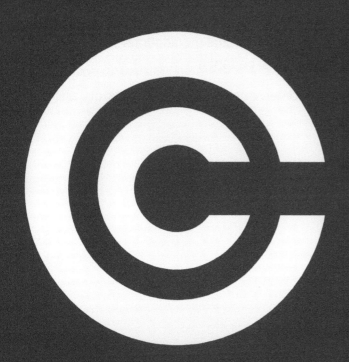

Small group session
Respiratory failure

Introduction

During this session, participants will follow the deteriorating course of a patient with respiratory failure.

Part 1 will consist of a brief discussion about the diagnosis and initial management of the hypoxic patient with special reference to the use of arterial blood gas results and ward-based ventilatory support such as continuous positive airway pressure (CPAP) and non-invasive ventilation (NIV).

Part 2 will enable the participant to learn basic airway skills and demonstrate these with the airway trainers.

Duration	25 minutes
Style	Group discussion and demonstration
Faculty	One or two, including at least one with anaesthetic skills
AV	NA

Resources

▶ 1.7.0 Arterial blood gas results for parts 1 and 2.

▶ 1.7.1 Non-invasive ventilation mask.

▶ 1.7.2 High-flow oxygen delivery system [high-flow nasal cannula (HFNC) or high-flow facemask (HFFM)].

▶ 1.7.3 Bag valve mask (BVM).

▶ 1.7.4 CPAP mask.

▶ BVM × 2.

▶ Airway trainer/manikin.

▶ Selection of oxygen masks, oral and nasopharyngeal airways.

▶ Suction equipment.

▶ Laryngeal mask airways (LMAs) sizes 3–5 and Endotracheal Tubes (ETs) sizes 7–9.

Learning outcomes

At the end of this session, participants will be able to:

▪ use the CCrISP system to recognise respiratory failure and institute basic airway management;

▪ recognise and state the difference between type 1 respiratory failure (hypoxaemia without hypercapnia) and type 2 respiratory failure (hypoxaemia with hypercapnia);

- establish and maintain airway patency and use the BVM;

- state indications for the use of non-invasive ventilatory support (CPAP and NIV). In some hospitals these services are ward based and surgical trainees may come across patients receiving NIV and there is likely to be increasing use of high-flow nasal cannula systems, eg Optiflow systems.

Teaching outline

Part 1

- In this session, participants will initially be asked to consider the clinical case of a patient with type 1 respiratory failure (hypoxaemia without hypercapnia) following aspiration and recognise this on an arterial blood gas analysis (ABG number 1).

- Discussion should concentrate on assessment of the patient's respiratory compromise using the CCrISP system. This should be limited to discussion of:

  - oxygen saturation

  - work of breathing (respiratory rate and use of accessory muscles)

  - chest auscultation for wheeze, crackles and loss of breath sounds.

- The use of the respiratory rate as a very important early indicator of critical illness should be stressed and related to the physiological need to increase oxygen uptake and to clear carbon dioxide in metabolic or respiratory acidosis.

- Discussion of the management in this part should be limited to the administration of high-flow mask oxygen using a rebreathe system, placing the patient in an upright position and the involvement of physiotherapy and critical care teams/outreach support.

- It may be appropriate to discuss ward-based ventilatory support such as CPAP and NIV to improve oxygenation and reduce the work of breathing. It should be stressed that such support is to be used only as a supportive measure while the underlying condition (wheeze, pulmonary oedema, collapse, infection) is treated and that prolonged use is inappropriate in a ward setting and may actually lead to patient harm. Photographs of CPAP, high-flow systems and NIV masks in use are provided within the teaching materials.

Part 2

- In part 2 the patient has deteriorated as a result of type 2 respiratory failure (hypercapnic hypoxaemia) and is now in need of airway support.

- This part of the session should initially present the patient as an acute airway emergency necessitating use of basic airway management skills. This should be manikin based and involve a graded approach to opening the airway and the use of the BVM.

- The session should start with a very brief presentation of ABG 2.

- All participants must have a chance to demonstrate basic airway skills.

- It is not appropriate for participants to attempt advanced airway management such as laryngeal mask insertion or intubation or the airway but they should all be aware that where basic management has failed these techniques will be required.

- The importance of calling promptly for urgent anaesthetic help must be stressed throughout.

Airway management teaching points

- Signs and types of respiratory failure.

- Use of diagnostic arterial blood gases.

- Patient positioning and oxygen.

- Use of ward-based ventilatory support.

- Signs of airway obstruction.

- Use of suctioning and removal of foreign bodies (including false teeth).

- Use of oral/nasopharyngeal airways.

- Bag valve mask ventilation.

- Calling for assistance.

Timeline

Introduction and objectives	2 minutes
Scenario 1	10 minutes
Scenario 2	10 minutes
Summary and questions	3 minutes

Scenario part 1

Brief to the participants

It is the weekend and you have been called to the ward by your foundation year 1 (FY1) to review an 82-year-old woman. She had an incisional hernia repair 2 days ago. She has had an episode of vomiting 2 hours previously and now her oxygen saturations are reading 88%. She is awake and talking but distressed and acutely short of breath.

The FY1 has performed an arterial blood gas (ABG 1) on air:

pH	7.42
PaO_2	7.6 kPa
$PaCO_2$	4.9 kPa
Base excess	−2 mmol/L
Lactate	1 mmol/L

Brief to faculty

This part of the scenario should take the form of a group discussion. Start by emphasising that candidates would do their own ABCDE assessment, which would help inform their planning. The candidates should recognise that the patient is in type 1 respiratory failure (hypoxaemia without hypercapnia) from the arterial blood gas.

Initial management should follow the CCrISP system and involve administration of oxygen and a brief examination of the patient's respiratory system.

A Intact.

B RR 25/min, is using accessory muscles and has coarse crackles and wheeze throughout her right lung field.

C No abnormalities.

D Alert but short of breath.

E No abnormalities.

The group should be asked for a brief management plan, which should include:

- following the rest of the CCrISP algorithm

- chest radiography

- physiotherapy

- referral to critical care/anaesthesia for consideration of ward-based (CPAP/NIV) ventilatory support or ventilatory support in a high-dependency unit.

In the final discussion participants should recognise that this is likely to represent aspiration pneumonitis.

Scenario part 2

This is a continuation of the scenario and can be used to introduce basic airway-opening manoeuvres and the correct assembly and use of the BVM. It is essential that all the participants have an opportunity to demonstrate basic airway skills on the manikin.

Brief to the participants

It is now 2 hours later and the patient was reviewed by a member of the critical care team, who instituted physiotherapy while organising a high-dependency bed. You have been urgently called back to the ward as the patient has become unresponsive and severely cyanosed. Prior to her collapse a blood gas was taken by your FY1 on 15 l/min oxygen:

ABG 2

pH	7.15
PaO_2	8.9 kPa
$PaCO_2$	9.2 kPa
Base excess	−4 mmol/L
Lactate	2.9 mmol/L

Brief to faculty

Start by telling the group a quick ABCDE assessment.

A Intact on oxygen.

B RR 15/min, otherwise unchanged chest signs.

C No change.

D Responds to voice.

E No change.

Start by asking the group to present ABG 2. This shows a type 2 respiratory failure (hypoxaemia with hypercapnia) and a **mixed** respiratory and metabolic acidosis. Make the point clearly that this links to the clinical findings of drop in RR and change in AVPU.

It may be useful to demonstrate the sequence below before asking each group member to manage the airway or ask one of the candidates to talk through and demonstrate while you check and correct if necessary.

Participants should be told that the oxygen mask is not fogging and should be asked in turn to manage the patient and should in order:

1. call for anaesthetic help with a cardiac arrest call;

2. open the airway with a chin lift and jaw thrust;

3. check for foreign bodies and suction the airway (the patient had vomited previously);

4. measure and appropriately demonstrate the insertion of both oral and nasal airways;

5. demonstrate correct assembly and use of the BVM (this can be a two-person task if necessary).

If time permits, a more advanced airway techniques can be discussed and demonstrated at this stage. **Participants should not be encouraged to practise advanced airway skills without significant experience**.

Key points

- Recognise and treat airway problems promptly to prevent cardiopulmonary arrest.

- Simple airway techniques will usually be best until skilled help arrives.

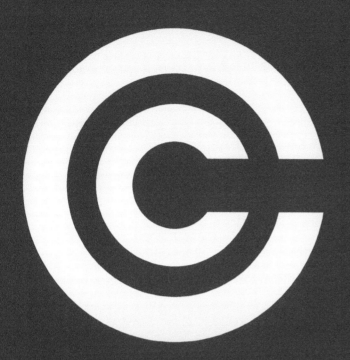

Small group session
Tracheostomy management

Introduction

During this session, participants learn about the three different types of tracheostomy insertion and features of the most commonly encountered tracheostomies and will be taught a simple algorithm for dealing with respiratory distress in a patient with a tracheostomy in situ.

Increasing numbers of patients are returning from intensive care and operating rooms with a tracheostomy in place. Surgical trainees are often unaware of the basics of tracheostomy management, and this session aims to redress this by concentrating on the basics required to appropriately manage the tracheostomy patient in distress.

Duration	25 minutes
Style	Group discussion and demonstration
Faculty	One or two, including at least one with anaesthetic/ENT skills
AV	NA

Resources

▶ 1.8.0 Learning objectives for the session and the participant brief including ABGs.

▶ 1.8.1 Types of tracheostomy and emergency tracheostomy management (patent upper airway) algorithm from the National Tracheostomy Safety Project (NTSP).

▶ 1.8.2 Lateral view of a laryngectomy and emergency laryngectomy management algorithm from the NTSP.

▶ 1.8.3 Trachi-pass courtesy of Kapitex Healthcare.

▶ 1.8.4 Tracheostomy in airway.

▶ Demonstration tracheostomies.

▶ Cuffed, unfenestrated with inner cannula × 2.

▶ Uncuffed fenestrated with fenestrated and unfenestrated inner cannulae.

Learning outcomes

At the end of this session, participants will be able to:

outline the clinical indications for the insertion of a tracheostomy;

outline the importance of recognising the difference between a tracheostomy and laryngectomy (end stoma tracheostomy) and how this relates to resuscitation strategies in these patient groups;

explain the difference between a surgical (slit or Bjork flap) and a percutaneous dilational tracheostomy;

identify the components of two forms of tracheostomy: a cuffed unfenestrated tracheostomy with an inner cannula and an uncuffed fenestrated tracheostomy with fenestrated and unfenestrated inner cannulae;

recognise the NTSP algorithm for emergency tracheostomy management with a patent upper airway.

Teaching outline

To ensure that the session keeps to time it is important that the structure is followed closely. The session should be interactive, a question and answer format works well.

Ensure learning objectives are outlined at the start.

The demonstrator starts by reviewing the indications for the insertion of a tracheostomy.

The demonstrator can then show the difference between a laryngectomy insertion (no patent upper airway) and a tracheostomy with a patent upper airway using the NTSP safety project laminated sheets provided and show the tracheostomy passports.

It must be emphasised that the lack of a patent upper airway in a laryngectomy patient rules out the use of facemask and upper airway devices in the event of respiratory distress.

On discussion of a tracheostomy in a patient with a patent upper airway, distinction must be made between surgical insertions (slit or Bjork flap), which make it likely that the stoma will remain open for some time following decannulation, and dilational percutaneous tracheostomies, which allow rapid stoma closure following tracheostomy removal.

The basics of tracheostomy care can be covered before moving on to the scenario.

If time permits, candidates should observe, handle and understand the main components of an uncuffed, fenestrated tracheostomy with a fenestrated cannula and unfenestrated inner cannula. They should understand that a fenestrated tracheostomy cannot be used to provide adequate bag ventilation because upper airway leak will be present in a non-laryngectomy patient without use of an unfenestrated inner cannula.

The final part of the session should follow a scenario format. The emphasis should be on ensuring that all the candidates understand the NTSP algorithm for hypoxia with a tracheostomy.

Part 1: Briefly review the indications for tracheostomy insertion

Upper airway obstruction.

Post-laryngectomy.

Risk of aspiration due to loss of upper airway reflexes.

- Minimise the risk of complications from long-term oral or nasal airway endotracheal intubation (reduces ventilator-associated pneumonia, oral secretions and sedation needs).

- Facilitate weaning from ventilation [decreases sedation needs, less airway resistance than with an endotracheal tube (ETT)].

- More effective airway toilet (easier access to deep lung suction, patient can cough more easily).

Part 2: Discuss the difference between laryngectomy with no patent upper airway and tracheostomy with a patent upper airway

- Use the laminated sheets and passport documents provided.

- It should be stressed that laryngectomy patients have no patent upper airway and therefore bag and facemask ventilation and LMA or ETT insertion is not an option if these patients develop respiratory distress. **Patients have died as a result of this not being appreciated by the resuscitating team.**

Part 3a: Cuffed unfenestrated tracheostomy with inner cannula

- Mainly used on ventilated patients in a critical care setting.

- During this section explain that the tracheostomy with cuff inflated forms a sealed airway to the lungs through which the patient can be effectively ventilated either mechanically or via a bag and valve ventilation system such as the AmbuBag. The cuff additionally protects against aspiration of upper airway contents.

- Demonstrate the cuff inflation and deflation process and mention briefly the dangers of overinflation (tracheal ischaemia and eventually stenosis).

- Use of the inner cannula to aid cleaning should also be discussed.

Part 3b: Uncuffed fenestrated tracheostomy with fenestrated and non-fenestrated inner cannulae

- This is used primarily in long-term tracheostomy patients, in whom the upper airway can be used for phonation. There is less protection from aspiration of upper airway contents.

- The fenestrated inner cannula allows for cleaning and the unfenestrated cannula can be used if bag and mask ventilation is required. Ventilation via an uncuffed tracheostomy will always be less effective than a cuffed tracheostomy.

Part 4: Tracheostomy care

It should be emphasised that all tracheostomies require a management package on a ward which should include:

- regular suction

- regular change of inner tube if applicable

- physiotherapy for secretion load

- patient and staff education

- bedside identifiers of the 'neck-breathing patient' where applicable.

Part 5: The National Tracheostomy Safety Project algorithm for emergency tracheostomy management with a patent upper airway

Using the NTSP algorithm on a laminated sheet and the cuffed unfenestrated tracheostomy with inner cannulae use the scenario below to discuss the management of the patient in respiratory distress with a tracheostomy in place.

Brief for the participant

You have been called by your foundation year 1 (FY1) to review a 68-year-old woman on the high-dependency unit. She had a ruptured abdominal aneurysm repair 14 days ago. Following this she required a percutaneous dilational tracheostomy for a respiratory wean and was on a spontaneous breathing mode (assisted spontaneous breathing/pressure support) on the ventilator and fully awake.

She has suddenly become distressed and acutely short of breath with saturations of 85% on 50% inspired oxygen concentration. Her capnography (expired CO_2) trace shows a very low expired CO_2 level from the tracheostomy.

The FY1 has performed an arterial blood gas on 50% O_2 with the following results:

pH	7.48
PaO_2	7.6 kPa
$PaCO_2$	3.1 kPa
Base excess	−1 mmol/L
Lactate	1 mmol/L

Brief for the instructor

This part of the scenario should take the form of a brief group discussion. Participants should recognise that the patient is in type 1 respiratory failure (hypoxaemia without hypercapnia) from the arterial blood gas and that the low capnography trace indicates an airway problem. If necessary the group should be guided to this diagnosis.

Initial management should follow the CCrISP system but be limited to airway management. This should follow the NTSP algorithm:

- Call for help.

- Recognise this is a patent upper airway case.

- Recognise that the patient is breathing but that this is suboptimal.

- Administer 100% oxygen via facemask and tracheostomy.

- Assess tracheostomy patency assessing for improving ventilation after each step:

    - remove inner cannula;

    - suction;

    - deflate cuff;

    - call for skilled assistance, eg anaesthetic or ICU support;

    - remove tracheostomy;

    - manage upper airway with bag mask ventilation + airway adjuncts;

    - attempt bag mask ventilation at tracheostomy stoma site;

    - intubate upper airway (it should be stressed that this should be done only by a clinician skilled at endotracheal intubation).

The demonstration tracheostomy should be used by each participant when assessing patency. This works best if the tracheostomy is passed from participant to participant asking 'what would you do next?' and requesting a demonstration of the step in question.

If possible, this should be done twice.

Summarise key points

- Relatively common on critical care and on specialist wards.

- Important to determine if the tracheostomy patient has a patent upper airway.

- Straightforward to manage with sufficient thought and knowledge of extant emergency algorithms.

- Seek help early.

- The upper airway can be successfully managed conventionally in most patients with tracheostomies.

Timeline

Introduction and objectives	2 minutes
Indications for tracheostomy use and the difference between a patient with a patent upper airway and a patient with a laryngectomy tracheostomy	7 minutes
Tracheostomy equipment and care	7 minutes
Scenario	9 minutes

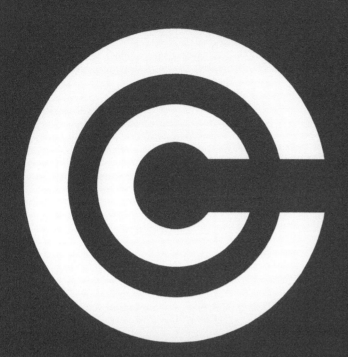

Small group session
Wound care

Introduction

In this session the participants will be given the opportunity to see and discuss various wounds and to discuss the management of wound infections, prevention of wound infections and the importance of necrotic tissue.

Duration	25 minutes
Style	Discussion groups of four participants
Faculty	One or two
AV	PowerPoint presentation

Learning outcomes

- To recognise and treat wound infection.

- To recognise and understand the significance of cellulitis and wound necrosis.

- To recognise an intestinal fistula and to describe the principles of management.

- To outline the principle of management of the open abdomen.

Teaching outline

Surgical trainees at this stage are often unsure how to assess or manage wounds. This can be an ideal session in which to draw on the experience of the nurse observers, who may have considerable experience of wound problems and management. Pictures are used to illustrate short scenarios.

It should be stressed at the start of the session that wound management is not always straightforward. In this session, the participants are taken through four scenarios that highlight important areas of wound management, including intestinal fistulae and the open abdomen. The whole group should be encouraged to be involved. Candidates are not expected to have extensive experience of the complexities of management of fistulae and the open abdomen and this element of the session is aimed more at knowledge transfer than at application of knowledge. To encourage group discussion it is suggested that the PowerPoint presentation should be used directly from a laptop rather than projected onto a screen.

Work through the objectives quickly, perhaps assessing the experience of the group in dealing with wounds, as this may vary considerably between participants. The first image (**slide 3**) is not related to a scenario but illustrates a normal laparotomy wound with a single abdominal drain. This should encourage a brief discussion about what features should be expected from a normal, non-infected wound and some basic aspects of drain management.

Leave time for questions and summarise at the end. The following four scenarios represent:

1. a wound abscess following an appendicectomy;

2. an infected, necrotic groin wound in an IV drug user that could be necrotising fasciitis;

3. a case of an intestinal fistula following incisional hernia repair without a prosthetic mesh;

4. a laparostomy following abdominal compartment syndrome.

Timeline

Introduction	2 minutes
Infection/wound abscess	4 minutes
Necrosis	4 minutes
Fistula	6 minutes
Open abdomen	6 minutes
Questions and summary	3 minutes

Resources

▶ Laptop.

Overview of scenarios

Scenario 1

You are asked to see a patient on the ward who underwent an open appendicectomy for a perforated, gangrenous appendix 4 days ago. He wants to go home but is complaining of pain in the wound. The nurses tell you he spiked a temperature of 38°C.

Discuss

▢ The features of wound infection and wound abscess (redness, swelling, heat and pain).

▢ The management of a wound abscess, including the role of abscess drainage and antibiotic therapy. Candidates may suggest flucloxacillin as this is mistakenly considered a skin-type infection – explain why this is wrong.

▢ The importance of antibiotic prophylaxis.

This is clearly a wound abscess following an appendicectomy. The general condition of the patient needs to be taken into consideration when deciding on management and the three-stage assessment process should be used to determine this. The abscess requires urgent incision and drainage. The second picture shows the incision of the abscess on the ward to drain the pus. Consideration should be given to this being performed in theatre so that a thorough wound exploration and lavage can be performed. Cultures should be taken to direct any further antibiotic therapy, but this is not the mainstay of treatment unless there is spreading cellulitis or systemic upset. Take the opportunity to discuss cellulitis both with and without underlying collections.

A senior member of the surgical team should be involved in the decision on how, when and where to treat wound infections/collections.

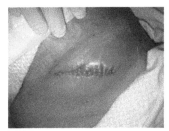

*(a) Obvious wound abscess without spreading cellulitis (**slide 5**).*

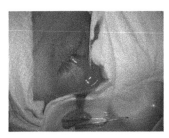

*(b) The wound is being drained on the ward: pus can be seen flowing from the wound into the receptacle (**slide 6**). The patient could now go to theatre for formal wound opening and lavage.*

Scenario 2

You are called to the emergency department to see a 34-year-old drug user with a tender swollen groin.

Discuss

- Assessing the patient systemically.

- Is the patient physiologically unstable?

- Is there evidence of false aneurysm?

- What is the risk of transmissible disease?

- Microbiology and synergistic necrotising infection.

Points to consider

- The patient may be septic and unstable – the participant should suggest assessment and simultaneous resuscitation using the CCrISP system of assessment.

- Consider microbiology advice but institute the Sepsis 6 including early IV antibiotics.

- This may require extensive debridement – consider the possibility of necrotising fasciitis but also the potential for an underlying false aneurysm.

- The patient could have an ultrasound scan prior to any debridement depending on availability and the time this will take.

- Also consider the risk of transmissible disease.

- A senior member of the team should be informed.

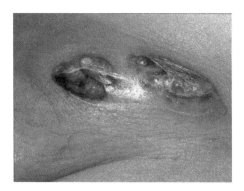

*Infected, necrotic groin wound (**slide 8**).*

Scenario 3

You are called to the ward to see a 60-year-old woman who has presented back to the ward 3 days after discharge following an incisional hernia repair for which she had an overnight stay. She had undergone a difficult incisional hernia repair, including extensive division of intra-abdominal adhesions. She initially felt OK after going home but subsequently became unwell. She developed a wound discharge, after which she felt a little better. Another doctor told her it was 'a bit of a wound infection'.

Discuss

- Intestinal fistulae: definitions, recognition and assessment.

- Assessment of the patient according to the CCrISP system of assessment.

- Management of fistulae by the SNAP(S) protocol:

  - sepsis (drain any collections, operate if peritonitis);

  - nutrition (what, when, how);

  - anatomy (delineate, when fit to do so);

  - procedure (reparative procedure when patient well, and only if fistula does not close spontaneously);

  - skin care.

Slide 12 gives the information in the order of the three-stage assessment process to encourage this approach and the patient's observations suggest relative stability. This means that immediate laparotomy should not be needed for control of sepsis and that a more considered approach can be taken.

▪ The wound has broken down and enteric contents are clearly visible in the lower wound.

▪ The immediate management must follow the CCrISP system. The management of the fistula can be discussed using the SNAP(S) protocol:

　• **Sepsis**. Manage sepsis by drainage of any collections; it may be necessary to perform computerised tomography (CT) then radiological or surgical drainage of any collections.

　• **Nutrition**. The patient will need nutritional support and this should be considered early. Any discussion about the pros and cons of enteral/parenteral nutrition in enteric fistulae should be brief, as these will be considered in more detail later in the course. Stress the importance of careful fluid/electrolyte balance in patients with fistulae. The patient should initially be nil by mouth. Output may be controllable medically.

　• **Anatomy**. Further investigations will be required to investigate the anatomy of the fistula, but this may be performed semi-electively. Discuss the roles of CT, contrast investigations, etc.

　• **Procedure**. A reparative procedure may be required at some point if the fistula fails to heal with conservative measures. The other complicating factor in this case is the incisional hernia repair. If a prosthetic mesh was used this may need to come out, and the surgical complexity is greater.

　• **Skin**. Skin can become macerated and damaged, especially if the fistula is discharging small bowel contents. Skin protection can be a major challenge.

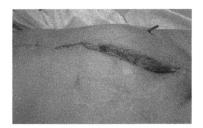

Slide 11

You are called to the intensive therapy unit (ITU) to see a patient who developed an abdominal compartment syndrome and necrotic colon after open repair of a ruptured abdominal aortic aneurysm. He had a Hartmann's procedure and laparostomy covered with a Vicryl mesh. The ITU staff are concerned about the appearance of the wound and the fluid loss from the mesh.

▪ Indications for laparostomy (damage control surgery, sepsis, abdominal compartment syndrome).

▪ Abdominal compartment syndrome and intra-abdominal hypertension including measurement of abdominal pressure and decompression.

Management of fluid and protein loss from the wound.

Skin care.

Risk of fistula formation.

Other methods of management (topical negative pressure, Bogota bag).

Timing of dressing change/relook and issues around closure (immediate or delayed).

Stoma care, which can be difficult with a laparostomy.

Points to consider

The wound and bowel look fine with no evidence of local sepsis or ischaemic bowel.

Fluid management and replacement is difficult but is helped by the use of a bowel or fluid collection bag.

The role of vacuum-assisted closure (VAC) in this situation may be discussed. There is some controversy about the best wound management strategy and timing of attempts to close the abdomen.

Care for the wound and stoma should be as meticulous as possible to prevent any contamination of the wound.

Early involvement of a plastic surgeon is often helpful. Longer term options include skin grafting and muscle release procedures.

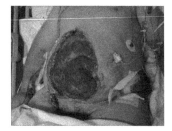

(a) Laparostomy: the bowel is covered with a Vicryl mesh (**slide 15**).
(b) Healed laparostomy following skin graft (**slide 18**).

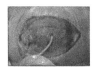

(c) VAC dressing in situ (**slide 17**).

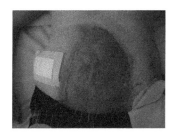

Summary

- Systematically assess the patient and wound.

- Drain any pus.

- Consider if antibiotics are indicated.

- Consider potential organisms and take microbiological advice.

- Recognise the specific situations of necrosis, fistulae and the open abdomen and seek appropriate support.

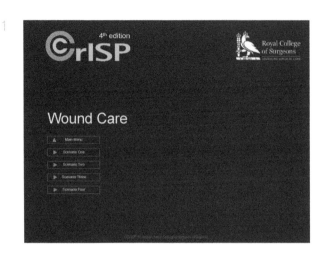

Learning Outcomes

- Recognise and treat wound infection
- Recognise and understand the significance of cellulitis and wound necrosis
- Describe how to recognise an intestinal fistula and the principles of fistula management
- Outline the management of the open abdomen

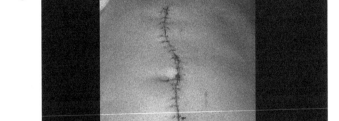

Scenario One

- You are asked to see a patient on the ward who underwent an open appendicectomy for a perforated, gangrenous appendicitis 4 days ago.
- He wants to go home but is complaining of pain in the wound.
- The nurses tell you he spiked a temperature of 38°C.

How will you assess this case?

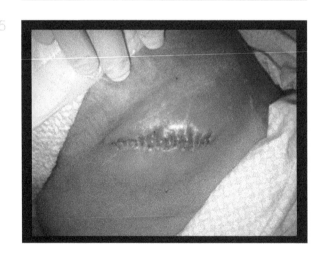

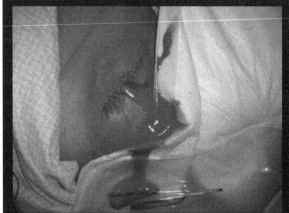

Use of antibiotics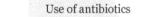

- Is there extensive cellulitis?
- Are there systemic symptoms?

Scenario Two

You are called to the emergency department to see a 34-year-old drug user with a tender and swollen groin.

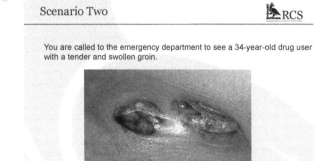

9
Scenario Two - summary

- Necrosis, including necrotising fasciitis is a potentially life threatening condition.
- Definitive treatment (surgical debridement) needs to be started as quickly as possible.

10
Scenario Three

- A 60-year-old lady presents back to the ward 3 days after discharge following an incisional hernia repair for which she had an overnight stay.
- She was initially OK but felt unwell after the second day at home.
- Today her wound discharged and she felt a little better.
- On initial assessment you find:
  - RR 22, P 110 reg, CRT 3 secs, BP 130/75, T 37.8°C
- The operation note shows that there were extensive intra-abdominal adhesions and mesh was not used.

11
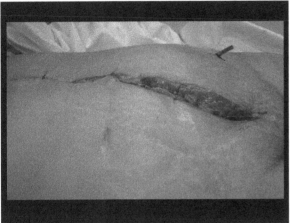

12
Scenario Three – Summary of management

- Assess/resuscitate the patient.
- SNAPS Protocol
  - Sepsis: assess and control sepsis
  - Nutrition: what, when and how to include fluid balance?
  - Anatomy: investigations to the level of the fistula
  - Procedure: decide if necessary, what will be done and when
  - Skin care: more of a problem with small bowel fistulae

13
Scenario Four

- You are called to ITU to see a patient who developed an abdominal compartment syndrome and necrotic colon after open repair of a ruptured abdominal aortic aneurysm.
- He had a Hartmann's procedure and laparostomy covered with a vicryl mesh.
- The ITU staff are concerned about the appearance of the wound and the fluid loss from the mesh.

14
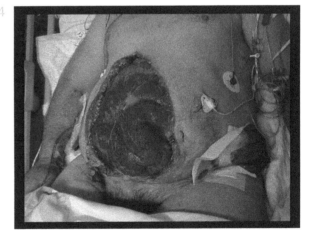

15
Considerations

- Indications for laparotomy:
  - Damage limitation surgery
  - Sepsis
  - Abdominal compartment syndrome
- Potential complications:
  - Heat and fluid loss
  - Protein loss
  - Skin care
    Fistula formation
- Issues to be dealt with:
  - Loss of domain, fascial retraction, subsequent closure

16
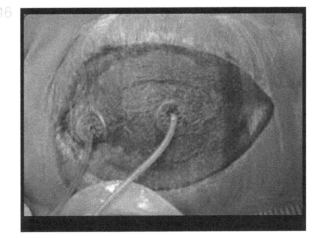

17

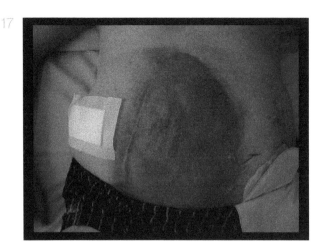

18

Any questions?

CC/riSP® 4ᵗʰ Edition Royal College of Surgeons of England

19

Summary

- Systematic assessment of the patient and wound.
- Drain any pus.
- Consider if antibiotics are indicated.
- Consider potential organisms and take microbiological advice.
- Recognise the specific situations of necrosis, fistulae and the open abdomen and seek appropriate support.

CC/riSP® 4ᵗʰ Edition Royal College of Surgeons of England

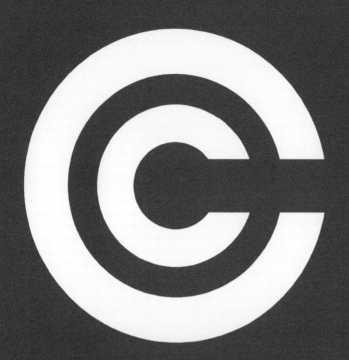

Small group session
Stoma care

Introduction

In this session the participants will be given the opportunity to see and discuss various stomas and to discuss the basic assessment and management of fistulas.

Duration	25 minutes
Style	Discussion groups of four students
Faculty	One or two
AV	PowerPoint presentation

Learning outcomes

1. Define different types of stoma and know how to assess them.

2. Assess a patient with stomas.

3. Recognise stomal complications.

Teaching outline

Surgical trainees are often unsure how to assess or manage stomas, though experience will vary greatly depending on their exposure to them on the wards. As with the wound session, this can be an ideal session in which to draw on the experience of the nurse observers, who may have considerable experience of stoma problems and management. Pictures in the PowerPoint presentation are used to illustrate short scenarios.

In this session, the candidates are introduced to stomas and an explanation of the different types and then are taken through scenarios that highlight important areas of stoma assessment and management, encouraging the whole group to be involved.

Work through the objectives quickly, perhaps assessing the experience of the group in dealing with stomas. The first photographs (**slides 3–6**) are not related to a scenario but illustrate a normal, healthy end colostomy, loop ileostomy and end ileostomy and show a classification of types of stomas. This should encourage a brief discussion about examples of when the different types of stomas may be used and what features and appearances should be expected from a normal stoma, together with some basic aspects of stoma management (skin care, appliances, etc). Ensure that candidates are aware that ill patients may deteriorate, particularly from sepsis, as a result of stoma complications. Patients should be assessed fully, using the CCrISP system of assessment.

Leave time for questions and summarise at the end. The following scenarios represent:

1. a dusky end colostomy, of dubious viability, in a stable patient who can be managed conservatively;

2. a necrotic end ileostomy and mucous fistula in an unstable patient who needs re-operation;

3. mucocutaneous separation, but otherwise healthy colostomy, in a stable patient.

The session is completed by going through some stomas which demonstrate the complications of:

 Stomal prolapse. Key to management is whether or not the bag can still be applied, stomal function and skin care. The condition can be managed conservatively. Revision is not always successful.

 Stenosis. Again management depends on function. Revision can be a major undertaking.

 Parastomal hernia. Management depends on symptoms, ability to apply the bag and function. Convex appliance and belt may help.

 Granulations. These can bleed. Consider silver nitrate or diathermy excision (which can be done under local anaesthesia).

 Retraction. Management depends on function and the ability to protect the skin. Convex appliance may help.

 Skin problems. These may be an allergic reaction or due to a poor-fitting appliance.

Involve the stoma nurse in dealing with complications.

Timeline

Introduction and objectives	2 minutes
Normal stomas, stoma care	4 minutes
Scenario 1: Patchy necrosis/assessment of viability	4 minutes
Scenario 2: Necrotic stoma	4 minutes
Scenario 3: Mucocutaneous separation	4 minutes
Stomal complications	4 minutes
Questions and summary	3 minutes

Resources

▶ Laptop.

▶ Optional: selection of stoma appliances/bags.

Overview of scenarios

Scenario 1

You are asked to see a patient on the HDU who underwent a Hartmann's procedure (end colostomy and closure of the rectal stump) 3 days ago. The nurses are concerned about the appearance of the stoma. The patient is otherwise well.

Discuss

- Assessment of the patient: a full assessment of the patient using the CCrISP system is required.

- Assessment of the stoma: the participants must have a clear understanding of how to examine a stoma thoroughly. They must do the following:

  - remove the bag;

  - look at the colour of the stoma and at any contents of the bag (in particular: Is the stoma functioning? Is there any blood?);

  - examine the skin around the stoma (for any discoloration or cellulitis or separation of the stoma from the skin);

  - perform digital examination of the stoma;

  - determine the extent of the discoloration of the stoma (participants need to know techniques for looking inside the stoma, such as the use of a disposable proctoscope or sigmoidoscope).

Points to consider

- This is an end colostomy with patchy necrosis, but there are areas of the stoma that appear viable.

- The management depends on the clinical status of the patient. In this case the patient is clinically improving and, after a thorough examination including assessment of the extent of the mucosal necrosis, a plan should be made to observe the patient.

- The patient and stoma should be checked regularly to ensure that neither has deteriorated.

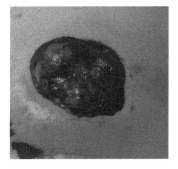

Slide 9

Scenario 2

You are called to the ICU to see a patient 3 days after a subtotal colectomy, ileostomy and mucous fistula for perforated ulcerative colitis. The patient is unstable and ICU staff are concerned about the stoma.

Discuss

- Assessment of the patient: a full assessment of the patient using the CCrISP system is required.

- The patient is septic and unwell, and therefore requires simultaneous resuscitation.

- The fact that stoma complications lead to systemic deterioration but that systemic illness can contribute to stoma complications.

- Assessment of the stoma.

- The difficulties that arise when assessing stomas, and the 'abdomen' as a whole, in the ICU setting.

Points

- The patient is septic and unstable – the participants should suggest assessment and simultaneous resuscitation using the CCrISP system of assessment.

- The stoma is non-viable and the mucous fistula is of dubious viability also, though this is difficult to see in the photo.

- Further observation will not change the management in this case and a plan should be made to return the patient to theatre for a further laparotomy urgently.

- A senior member of the team should be informed immediately.

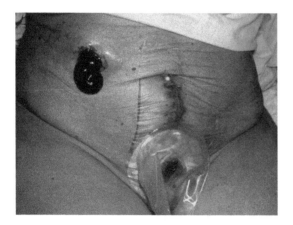

Slide 12

Scenario 3

On the morning ward round, a 74-year-old man, 10 days post Hartmann's procedure, asks if he can go home. He is doing well clinically. You decide to examine the stoma before authorising his discharge.

Discuss

- Mucocutaneous separation.

- Assessment of stoma and stoma function.

- Local wound management/cleaning and skin care.

- Stoma nurse input.

Points to consider

- The candidates should assess the whole patient prior to discharge. This should include a systematic examination and stoma examination, ensuring that the patient is able to care for the stoma and that adequate social support is in place.

- Mucocutaneous separation is relatively common but rarely causes any problems. The stoma looks healthy and is clearly working, and although there is some slough and overgranulation this is of little concern in a healthy patient ready for discharge. The stoma should still be examined carefully to ensure that there is no fistula. The key point is recognising that this is not a major problem and understanding the importance of local wound/skin care, and careful management by stoma/community nurses. Appropriate review in the community or review at the hospital should be suggested.

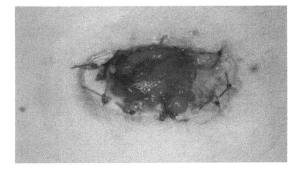

Slide 15

The stoma in scenario 3 is a complication of stoma formation and this leads us on to other complications. Some discussion points are given above and some of the possible causes of the complications can also be explored if there is time.

Summary

- Systematic assessment of the patient and stoma.

- Is the stoma viable?

- If unsure, get help and/or reassess.

- Stoma function, ability to fit the appliance and careful symptomatic assessment determines management of longer term complications.

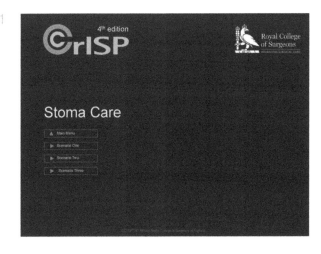

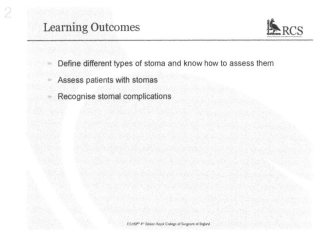

Learning Outcomes

- Define different types of stoma and know how to assess them
- Assess patients with stomas
- Recognise stomal complications

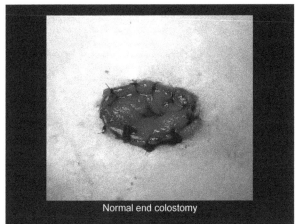

Normal end colostomy

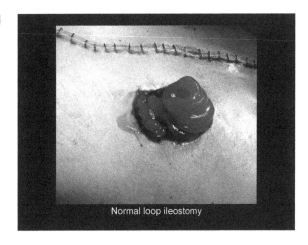

Normal loop ileostomy

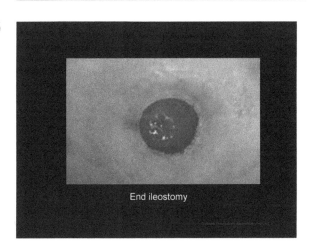

End ileostomy

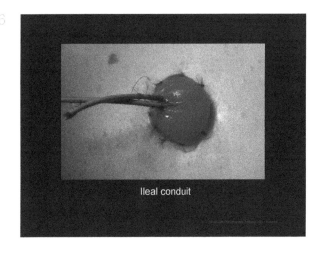

Ileal conduit

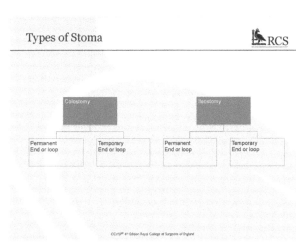

Types of Stoma

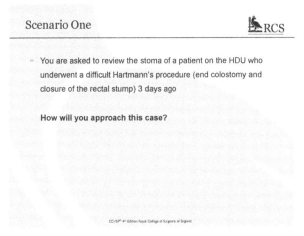

Scenario One

- You are asked to review the stoma of a patient on the HDU who underwent a difficult Hartmann's procedure (end colostomy and closure of the rectal stump) 3 days ago

How will you approach this case?

9

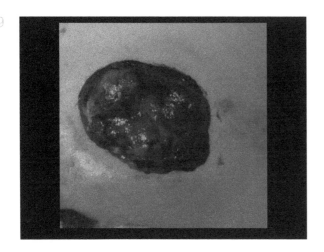

10

11

Scenario Two

- You are called to the ICU to see a patient 3 days after a subtotal colectomy, ileostomy and mucous fistula performed for perforated ulcerative colitis.
- The nurses tell you the patients BP has been difficult to maintain, the urine output is poor and the patient is now requiring inotropes.

CCrISP 4ᵗʰ Edition Royal College of Surgeons of England

12

13

Scenario Two – summary

- Definitive treatment is laparotomy and refashioning of the stoma.
- Liaise with ICU staff to optimise the patient's condition.
- Liaise with appropriate senior to confirm the plan and to decide on timing of surgery.

CCrISP 4ᵗʰ Edition Royal College of Surgeons of England

14

Scenario Three

- On the morning ward round, a 74-year-old man, 10 days post Hartmann's procedure, asks if he can go home.
- He is doing well clinically.
- The nurse has taken the stoma bag off and asks you to look at the stoma.

CCrISP 4ᵗʰ Edition Royal College of Surgeons of England

15

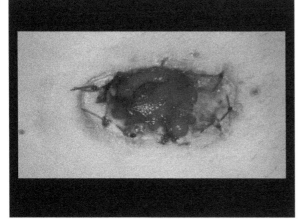

16

Scenario Three - Summary

- The stoma is healthy, as is the surrounding skin.
- It is functioning.
- There is a small amount of slough to one side and over-granulation, but this is of no great concern.
- Discharge of the patient with appropriate support and clinical review is appropriate.

What are the possible long term complications of a stoma?

CCrISP 4ᵗʰ Edition Royal College of Surgeons of England

17

Some stomal complications

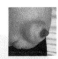RCS

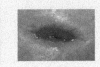

Stomal Prolapse

Stomal Stenosis

Parastomal Hernia

Stomal Granulations

Stomal Retraction

Stoma related skin excoriation

CCrISP® 4ᵗʰ Edition Royal College of Surgeons of England

18

RCS

Any questions?

CCrISP® 4ᵗʰ Edition Royal College of Surgeons of England

19

Summary

RCS

- Use the 3 stage assessment to evaluate the patient and include the stoma in E or full patient assessment.
- Assess stomal viability and function.
- Know where to get further help and advice from.

CCrISP® 4ᵗʰ Edition Royal College of Surgeons of England

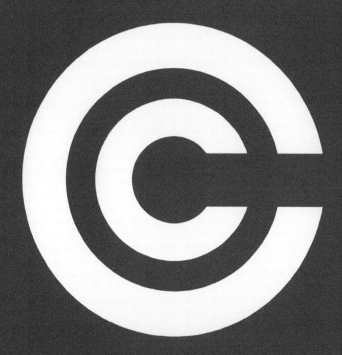

Small group session

Perioperative cardiac disorders

Introduction

During this session, participants will discuss the management of atrial fibrillation (AF) and acute coronary syndrome as two of the commonest perioperative cardiac disorders they are likely to come across.

The aim of the session is for them to gain an understanding of their role in assessing and treating these problems, not to teach participants everything about the ECG or managing cardiac problems.

The session starts with an overview of the types of perioperative cardiac problems trainees may come across, followed by a brief review of a technique for reading the ECG. The major part of the session deals with two patient scenarios, one of AF that degrades to ventricular tachycardia (VT) and ventricular fibrillation (VF), and a second case of a patient developing an acute anterior myocardial infarction (MI) after endovascular aneurysm repair.

Duration	45 minutes
Style	Group discussion and demonstration
Faculty	One or two, including at least one with anaesthetic/ICU skills
AV	PowerPoint presentation

Resources

▶ Flipchart.

▶ Laptop.

Learning outcomes

At the end of this session, participants will be able to:

- use the ECG as part of the systematic approach to patient assessment;

- interpret and outline a simple treatment plan for common perioperative cardiac and rhythm problems;

- describe the methods of preoperative preparation and risk prediction.

Teaching outline

Slide 3 familiarises participants with the types of cardiac problems they may come across in the perioperative period. Make the point that many of them will respond to first-line treatments and stress the importance of appropriate patient assessment.

Slides 4 and **5** should not be laboured but provide a brief reminder of an approach to reading an ECG.

Slides 6 and **7** introduce a patient with new-onset AF. **Slide 8** illustrates two different rhythm strips on the monitor and links them to the patient parameters below.

Slide 10 indicates the importance of conducting the second-stage full patient assessment and chart review correctly as this allows simple treatments as well as helping to determine the possible cause.

Slide 12 shows that the patient's BP has now fallen, which makes treatment of the AF more urgent. This leads into **slide 13**, which illustrates some of the key treatment options and makes the point that anticoagulation is often undesirable in the acute surgical patient. Candidates can be referred to NICE guidelines on assessing the risk of stroke in patients with AF, which is outside the remit of this course.

Slide 14 is the American College of Cardiology decision tree for acute onset of AF and should be shown to make the point that a full patient assessment is needed in new-onset AF to rule out a surgical cause and help determine the medical options for further treatment.

Slides 15–18 introduce a new case of a patient developing chest pain 3 days after endovascular aneurysm repair.

Slides 19 and **20** introduce the types of preoperative cardiac assessment that this patient, as a known arteriopath, may have had. Make the point that looking for this preoperative information as part of the chart review will provide valuable information to help guide current management.

Slides 22 and **23** show the monitor and ECG appearances of an acute ST segment elevation consistent with an acute anterior MI.

Slide 24 shows that an acute MI in the perioperative period is a significant problem and management must involve discussion at senior medical and surgical levels. The treatment of choice in an interventional centre would be an urgent percutaneous coronary intervention (PCI). NICE recommends that in adults with acute ST segment elevation MI (STEMI) who present within 12 hours of onset of symptoms the preferred coronary reperfusion strategy is PCI, which should be performed as soon as possible, but in any event within 120 minutes of the time when fibrinolysis could have been given.

Slides 25 and **26** indicate acute VT and treatment options. VT degrades quickly to VF in **slide 27**.

Slides 30–34 should not be introduced after the summary slides but, if there is time, can be used to take candidates through some additional clinical material prior to finishing with the questions and summary **slides 28** and **29**:

- **Slide 30** shows sinus bradycardia with a low BP secondary to beta blockade. Heart rate cannot be increased to raise cardiac output and BP. This can compromise the response to hypovolaemia so attention to fluid balance is important.

- **Slide 31** shows multiple, frequent ventricular ectopics. These are not normal and should be investigated. In the post-surgical patient, electrolyte imbalance is the commonest cause (eg potassium and magnesium abnormalities). Untreated they may lead to more serious cardiac dysrhythmias.

- **Slide 32** shows AF with reasonably slow rate. This will require continued treatment if already diagnosed or referral to cardiology if new onset.

- **Slide 33** shows left bundle branch block, which is always pathological and indicates underlying cardiac disease.

- **Slide 34** shows a paced rhythm which will require a pacemaker check preoperatively. In patients with pacemakers and implantable cardiac defibrillators (ICDs), it is necessary to consult with the cardiac physiology department before surgery.

Timeline

Introduction and objectives	3 minutes
Cardiac disorders and ECG review	5 minutes
Scenario 1	15 minutes
Scenario 2	20 minutes
Questions and summary	2 minutes

1

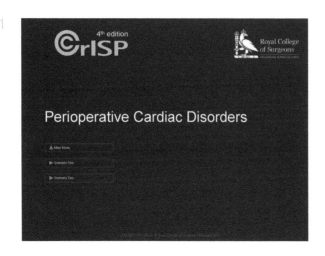

2

Objectives

- Use the ECG as part of the systematic approach to patient assessment.
- Interpret common peri-operative cardiac and rhythm problems.
- Outline a simple treatment plan for common peri-operative cardiac and rhythm problems
- Describe the methods of pre-operative preparation and risk prediction.

CCrISP® 4th edition © Royal College of Surgeons of England 2017

3

Common post-op cardiac disorders

What common cardiac problems do you see in peri-operative patients?

- Atrial fibrillation.
- Ischaemia and infarction.
- Tachycardia, to increase cardiac output in response to bleeding, hypovolaemia or sepsis.
- Be aware of medication that will mask hypovolemia and compensatory tachycardia. i.e. beta blockers, ACEI
- Cardiac failure as a consequence of one of the above, very occasionally iatrogenic fluid overload.
- The ECG can help with diagnosis and treatment.

CCrISP® 4th edition © Royal College of Surgeons of England 2017

4

Reading a 12 lead ECG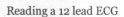

- Rate
- Rhythm
- P waves: presence and relation to QRS
- PR interval
- Width of QRS complex
- QRS and T wave duration and morphology

CCrISP® 4th edition © Royal College of Surgeons of England 2017

5

CCrISP® 4th edition © Royal College of Surgeons of England 2017

6

Scenario One

- You are called to see a 74-year-old man on the surgical ward.
- 3 days post-op low anterior resection.
- You are asked to see him as he is tachycardic and hypotensive.

What would you do?

CCrISP® 4th edition © Royal College of Surgeons of England 2017

7

Scenario one: immediate management

- **A** Patient speaking. Give high flow oxygen
- **B** Clear
- **C** HR 120, BP 100/70 mmHg
- **D** Alert
- **E** Awaiting full exam

CCrISP® 4th edition © Royal College of Surgeons of England 2017

8

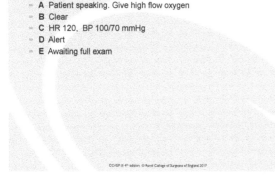

9

What else do you want to check in the full patient assessment and chart review?

10

Scenario one: treatment

RCS

- Is the patient hypovolaemic?
- breathlessness/dyspnoea?
- Palpitations?
- syncope/dizziness?
- chest discomfort?
- stroke/transient ischaemic attack?
- Oxygen
- K⁺, Mg²⁺
- Any drug omissions? Chronic AF?
- Any surgical cause? Sepsis/bleeding
- Any other underlying cause? PE, MI, thyroid
- Is the patient stable or unstable?

11

Scenario one: progress

RCS

You are called back to see the patient because his blood pressure has dropped.

How would you manage the situation?

Reassess using the CCrISP 3 stage assessment

12

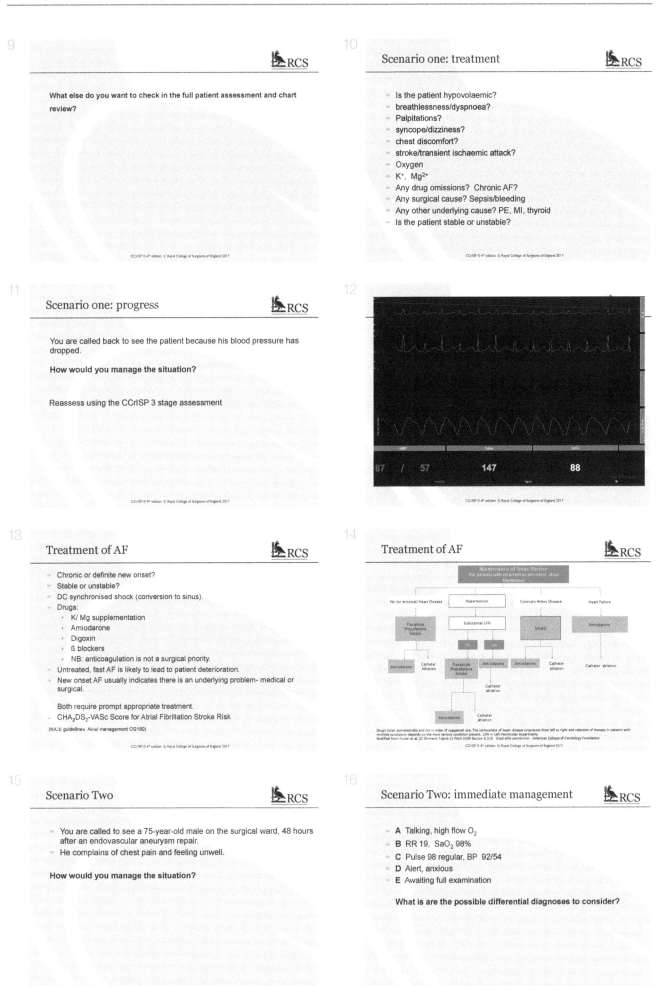

13

Treatment of AF

RCS

- Chronic or definite new onset?
- Stable or unstable?
- DC synchronised shock (conversion to sinus).
- Drugs:
  - K/ Mg supplementation
  - Amiodarone
  - Digoxin
  - ß blockers
  - NB: anticoagulation is not a surgical priority.
- Untreated, fast AF is likely to lead to patient deterioration.
- New onset AF usually indicates there is an underlying problem- medical or surgical.

  Both require prompt appropriate treatment.
- CHA₂DS₂-VASc Score for Atrial Fibrillation Stroke Risk

(NICE guidelines. Atrial management CG180)

14

Treatment of AF

RCS

15

Scenario Two

RCS

- You are called to see a 75-year-old male on the surgical ward, 48 hours after an endovascular aneurysm repair.
- He complains of chest pain and feeling unwell.

How would you manage the situation?

16

Scenario Two: immediate management

RCS

- **A** Talking, high flow O₂
- **B** RR 19, SaO₂ 98%
- **C** Pulse 98 regular, BP 92/54
- **D** Alert, anxious
- **E** Awaiting full examination

What is are the possible differential diagnoses to consider?

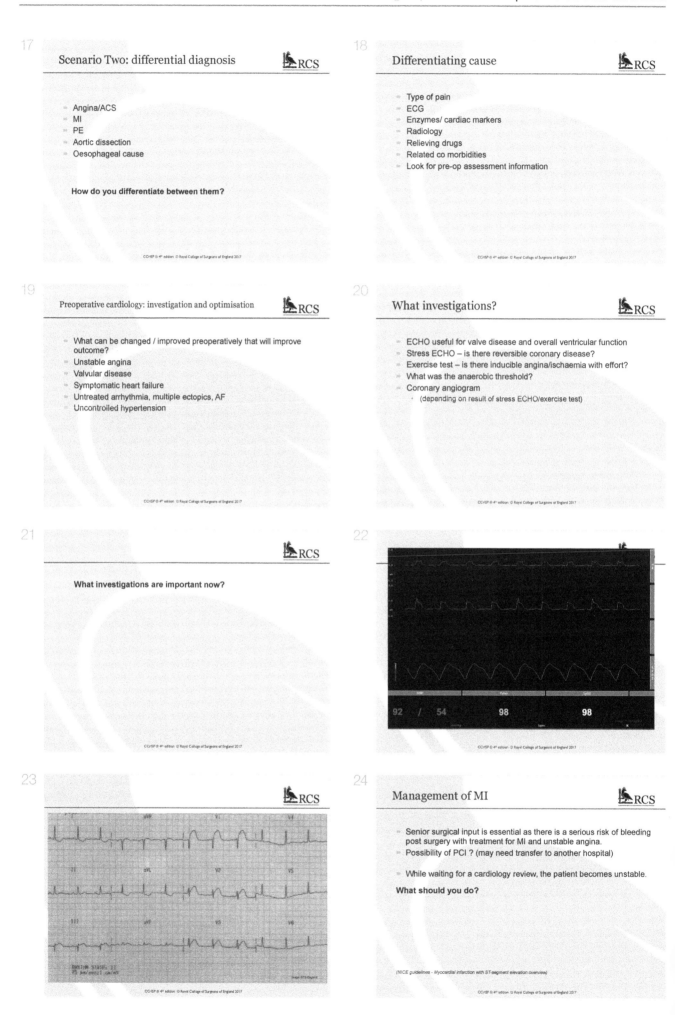

Slide 17

Scenario Two: differential diagnosis

- Angina/ACS
- MI
- PE
- Aortic dissection
- Oesophageal cause

How do you differentiate between them?

Slide 18

Differentiating cause

- Type of pain
- ECG
- Enzymes/ cardiac markers
- Radiology
- Relieving drugs
- Related co morbidities
- Look for pre-op assessment information

Slide 19

Preoperative cardiology: investigation and optimisation

- What can be changed / improved preoperatively that will improve outcome?
- Unstable angina
- Valvular disease
- Symptomatic heart failure
- Untreated arrhythmia, multiple ectopics, AF
- Uncontrolled hypertension

Slide 20

What investigations?

- ECHO useful for valve disease and overall ventricular function
- Stress ECHO – is there reversible coronary disease?
- Exercise test – is there inducible angina/ischaemia with effort?
- What was the anaerobic threshold?
- Coronary angiogram
  - (depending on result of stress ECHO/exercise test)

Slide 21

What investigations are important now?

Slide 22

92 / 54   98   98

Slide 23

Slide 24

Management of MI

- Senior surgical input is essential as there is a serious risk of bleeding post surgery with treatment for MI and unstable angina.
- Possibility of PCI ? (may need transfer to another hospital)
- While waiting for a cardiology review, the patient becomes unstable.

What should you do?

(NICE guidelines - Myocardial infarction with ST-segment elevation overview)

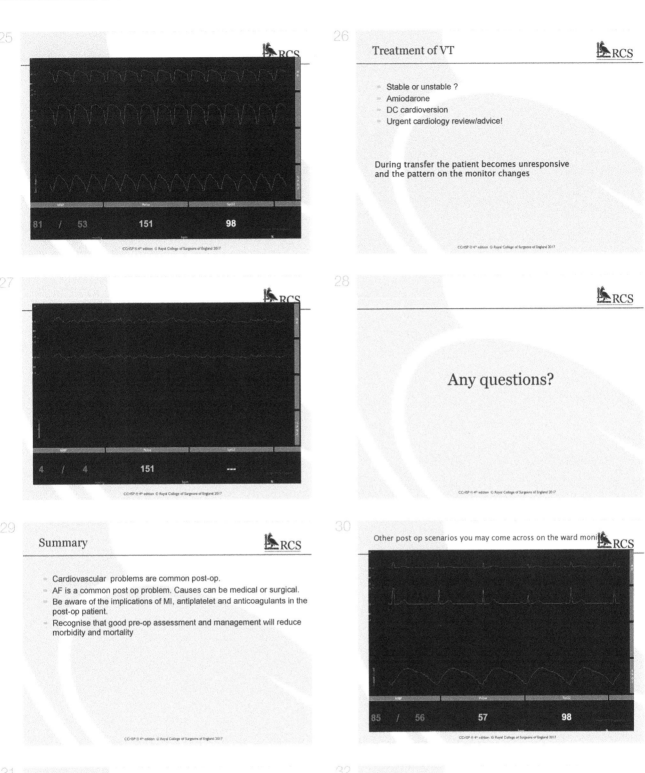

26

Treatment of VT

- Stable or unstable ?
- Amiodarone
- DC cardioversion
- Urgent cardiology review/advice!

During transfer the patient becomes unresponsive and the pattern on the monitor changes

28

Any questions?

29

Summary

- Cardiovascular problems are common post-op.
- AF is a common post op problem. Causes can be medical or surgical.
- Be aware of the implications of MI, antiplatelet and anticoagulants in the post-op patient.
- Recognise that good pre-op assessment and management will reduce morbidity and mortality

30

Other post op scenarios you may come across on the ward monitor

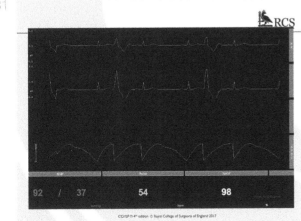

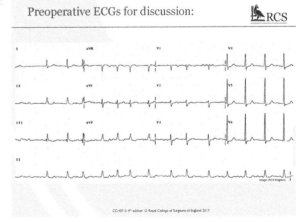

32

Preoperative ECGs for discussion:

33

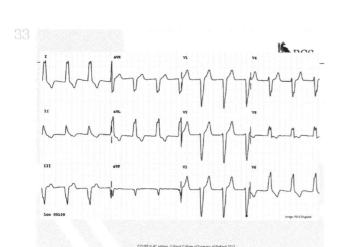

34

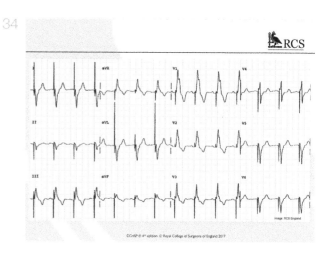

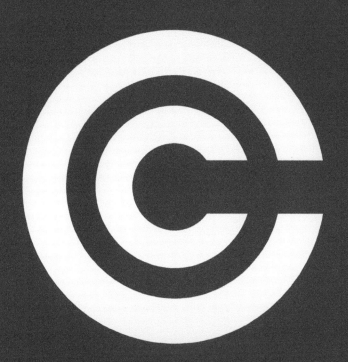

Small group session
Cardiovascular manipulation in shock

The aim of this session is to correlate the clinical management of a patient with underlying physiological principles and uses a case of severe pancreatitis to illustrate this. The slides are animated to aid the running of the session but these can be changed to suit individual faculty.

Learning outcomes

At the end of this session, participants will be able to:

- review the clinical management of shock in acutely unwell patients;

- establish the relationships between the physiological variables that can be manipulated in shock;

- illustrate how physiological changes relate to clinical management of the acutely unwell patient.

Resources

▶ Laptop.

▶ PowerPoint presentation.

Timeline

Introduction and learning outcomes	2 minutes
Main session	36 minutes
Questions	5 minutes
Summary	2 minutes

Teaching outline

Slide 3 introduces the case of a 40-year-old man who will turn out to have pancreatitis with marked physiological disturbance at presentation that responds only partly to resuscitation with oxygen and fluids and who is referred to the critical care service.

Slide 4 shows the findings on the initial patient assessment and asks whether the patient is shocked, the answer to which is 'yes' on the basis of the prolonged capillary refill time (CRT), the tachycardia and the low blood pressure.

Slide 5 explores the definition of shock and the fact that it can be managed using the three-stage assessment process to support the abnormal physiology while the underlying cause is determined and a definitive management plan formulated. The aim of treatment is to optimise oxygen delivery by giving oxygen at 15 L/min and by improving cardiac output with fluid challenges. The cardiac output side of this is addressed first, followed by other ways to manipulate oxygen delivery, such as ensuring adequate haemoglobin levels and ensuring that there are no ventilation–perfusion mismatches.

Slide 6 is a diagrammatic representation of the circulation and can be used to illustrate the point that the only part of the circulation we can easily monitor is the systemic arteries.

Slides 7–9 relate the physiology of cardiac output to blood pressure and link cardiac output to Starling's law of the heart. The graphic shows stroke volume (SV) plotted against left ventricular end-diastolic volume (LVEDV). It is worth relating these to surrogates of these axes; LVEDV relates to preload and venous filling and SV relates to CO and CRT, the latter being a useful sign when assessing the results of a fluid challenge and one that can give some indication of where the patient is on the Starling curve. In this way a fluid challenge can be considered to be diagnostic as well as therapeutic. Discussing the time course of the physiological response to a fluid challenge can help relate the physiology to what is done in clinical practice (changes in CRT, heart rate and blood pressure are more rapid than changes in urine output, for example). Furthermore, patients' responses depend on their cardiovascular reactivity and physiological reserve, and these factors need to be taken into account when evaluating a patient's physiological status.

Although tachycardia is a normal response to shock, for the reasons stated above, it may not always be possible for a patient to mount a tachycardia and a prolonged tachycardia may be undesirable because of its effects on cardiac oxygen requirements and oxygen availability.

Slide 10 introduces oxygen delivery, the manipulation of which is then explained in more detail in slides 16–22.

Slides 11–13 return to the scenario, when it becomes apparent that the diagnosis is pancreatitis. Given the abnormal physiology, sepsis should be considered as a cause, and it may be worth having some discussion around this. The patient's Quick Sequential Organ Failure Assessment (qSOFA)) score is 2, but there is no evidence of an infection. However, some candidates may want to perform the Sepsis 6, which is appropriate, and give antibiotics even though there is no definite indication for these in the initial management of pancreatitis. The 2016 NCEPOD report *Treat The Cause* describes the effects of inappropriate use of antibiotics in acute pancreatitis and candidates could be directed to read this report at a later date.

The abnormal blood glucose level should be noted by the candidates and this should be controlled with a variable-rate insulin infusion.

Slides 14 and **15** are a reminder of the stage in the assessment process that has been reached. The patient is unstable at present but may respond to resuscitation – this is yet to be determined by reassessment after the initial treatment.

Slides 16–22 explain oxygen delivery in more detail. The purpose of the oxygen–haemoglobin dissociation curve is to relate SaO_2 in the equation to FiO_2, which is the variable that is directly manipulated.

Slides 23–26 return to the scenario for the reassessment of the patient after 3 hours of treatment and show that the patient remains unstable after a significant amount of resuscitation, indicating the need for referral for a critical care opinion. Candidates should interpret the data, form a view of the overall situation and draw up a plan to refer the patient for a higher level of care.

Slide 27 shows what critical care services can offer and candidates should be clear about the reasons for referral to critical care and **slides 28** and **29** show how the adequacy of the treatment can be monitored using central venous oxygen saturations. Measuring central venous oxygen saturation is a now a common proxy for mixed venous oxygen saturations as the use of pulmonary artery catheters has declined. It is an indicator of the degree of adequacy of oxygen delivery and uptake by the tissues.

Slide 30 questions.

Slide 31 summary.

1

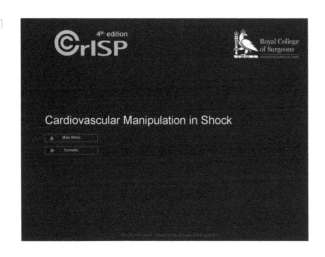

4th edition
CrISP

Royal College
of Surgeons

Cardiovascular Manipulation in Shock

Main Menu

Scenario

2

Objectives

- Review the clinical management of shock in acutely unwell patients
- Establish the relationships between the physiological variables that can be manipulated in shock
- Illustrate how physiological changes relate to clinical management of the acutely unwell patient

CCrISP ® 4th edition © Royal College of Surgeons of England 2017

3

Case Discussion

- 40 year old Somali man
- 2 month history of upper abdominal pain, acutely worse prior to admission.
- Epigastric pain with no radiation and associated with vomiting.
- No fever and no history of alcohol use.

CCrISP ® 4th edition © Royal College of Surgeons of England 2017

4

CCrISP 1st stage assessment

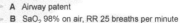

- **A** Airway patent
- **B** SaO_2 98% on air, RR 25 breaths per minute
- **C** P120 regular, CRT 5s, BP 75/50mmHg
- **D** Alert
- **E** Marked abdominal pain. Epigastric tenderness and no guarding.

Is this man shocked?

CCrISP ® 4th edition © Royal College of Surgeons of England 2017

5

Shock

What is shock?

- Shock is an acute circulatory failure leading to inadequate perfusion, acute cellular hypoxia and cell death

How do we assess and treat shock?

- Oxygen 15l/minute and fluid challenge in 1st stage assessment
- complete 3 stage assessment for possible causes and to decide and plan appropriately
- further treatment depends on cause

CCrISP ® 4th edition © Royal College of Surgeons of England 2017

6

CCrISP ® 4th edition © Royal College of Surgeons of England 2017

7

What determines cardiac output?

Cardiac Output = Heart rate x Stroke Volume

- Typically,
- Cardiac Output = 70 beats per minute x 70 mls per beat or 4,900 mls blood/minute i.e. 5 litres/minute
- In shock, one normal physiological response is to increase heart rate to maintain cardiac output

CCrISP ® 4th edition © Royal College of Surgeons of England 2017

8

Cardiac output

- BP = CO x SVR
- CO = SV x HR, thus BP = SV x HR x SVR
- SV determined by
  - preload (Starling's Law)
  - contractility
  - afterload

CCrISP ® 4th edition © Royal College of Surgeons of England 2017

9

Starling curve

RCS

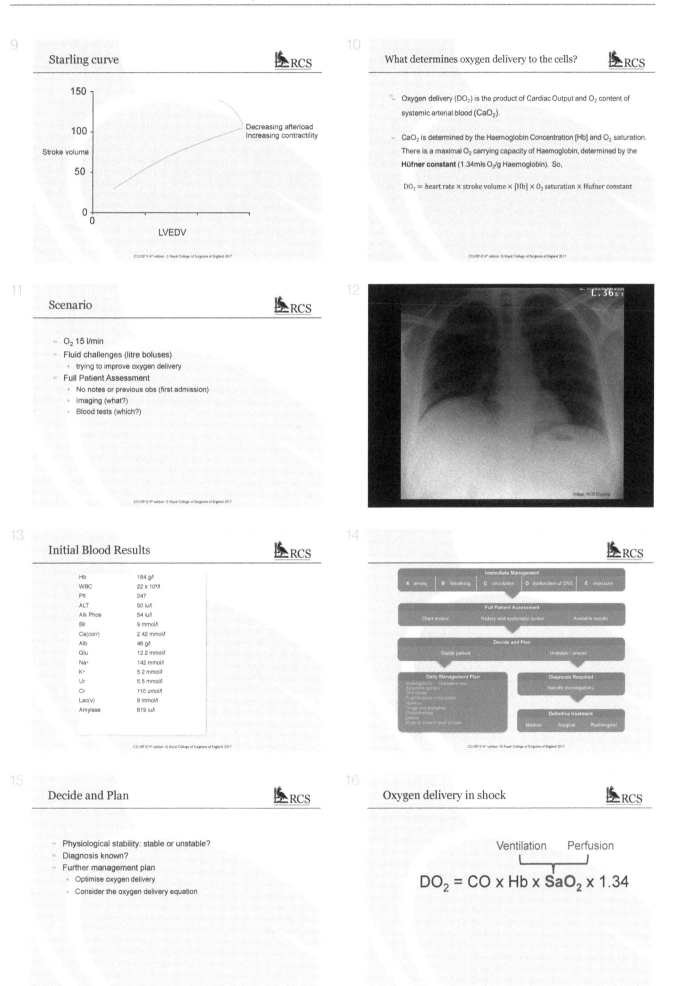

Stroke volume

150

100

50

0

0

LVEDV

Decreasing afterload
Increasing contractility

CCrISP ® 4ᵗʰ edition © Royal College of Surgeons of England 2017

10

What determines oxygen delivery to the cells?

RCS

- Oxygen delivery (DO_2) is the product of Cardiac Output and O_2 content of systemic arterial blood (CaO_2).

- CaO_2 is determined by the Haemoglobin Concentration [Hb] and O_2 saturation. There is a maximal O_2 carrying capacity of Haemoglobin, determined by the **Hüfner constant** (1.34mls O_2/g Haemoglobin). So,

$$DO_2 = \text{heart rate} \times \text{stroke volume} \times [Hb] \times O_2 \text{ saturation} \times \text{Hufner constant}$$

CCrISP ® 4ᵗʰ edition © Royal College of Surgeons of England 2017

11

Scenario

RCS

- O_2 15 l/min
- Fluid challenges (litre boluses)
  - trying to improve oxygen delivery
- Full Patient Assessment
  - No notes or previous obs (first admission)
  - Imaging (what?)
  - Blood tests (which?)

CCrISP ® 4ᵗʰ edition © Royal College of Surgeons of England 2017

12

L. 36

Image: RCS England

13

Initial Blood Results

RCS

Hb	184 g/l
WBC	22 x 10⁹/l
Plt	247
ALT	50 iu/l
Alk Phos	54 iu/l
Bil	9 mmol/l
Ca(corr)	2.42 mmol/l
Alb	46 g/l
Glu	12.2 mmol/l
Na⁺	142 mmol/l
K⁺	5.2 mmol/l
Ur	5.5 mmol/l
Cr	110 umol/l
Lac(v)	9 mmol/l
Amylase	619 iu/l

CCrISP ® 4ᵗʰ edition © Royal College of Surgeons of England 2017

14

RCS

Immediate Management

| A airway | B breathing | C circulation | D dysfunction of CNS | E exposure |

Full Patient Assessment

Chart review — History and systematic review — Available results

Decide and Plan

Stable patient — Unstable / unsure

Daily Management Plan
Investigations
Specialist opinion
Oral intake
Fluid balance prescription
Nutrition
Drugs and analgesia
Physiotherapy
Drains
Move to a lower level of care

Diagnosis Required
Specific investigations

Definitive treatment
Medical — Surgical — Radiological

CCrISP ® 4ᵗʰ edition © Royal College of Surgeons of England 2017

15

Decide and Plan

RCS

- Physiological stability: stable or unstable?
- Diagnosis known?
- Further management plan
  - Optimise oxygen delivery
  - Consider the oxygen delivery equation

CCrISP ® 4ᵗʰ edition © Royal College of Surgeons of England 2017

16

Oxygen delivery in shock

RCS

Ventilation   Perfusion

$$DO_2 = CO \times Hb \times SaO_2 \times 1.34$$

CCrISP ® 4ᵗʰ edition © Royal College of Surgeons of England 2017

17
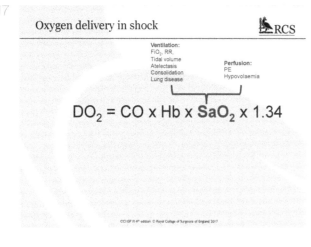

Oxygen delivery in shock

Ventilation:
FiO$_2$, RR,
Tidal volume
Atelectasis
Consolidation
Lung disease

Perfusion:
PE
Hypovolaemia

$$DO_2 = CO \times Hb \times SaO_2 \times 1.34$$

18
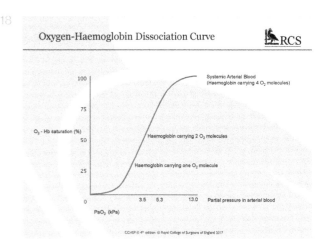

Oxygen-Haemoglobin Dissociation Curve

19
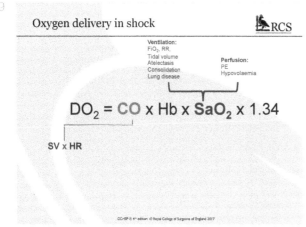

Oxygen delivery in shock

Ventilation:
FiO$_2$, RR,
Tidal volume
Atelectasis
Consolidation
Lung disease

Perfusion:
PE
Hypovolaemia

$$DO_2 = CO \times Hb \times SaO_2 \times 1.34$$

SV x HR

20
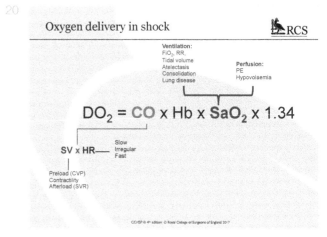

Oxygen delivery in shock

Ventilation:
FiO$_2$, RR,
Tidal volume
Atelectasis
Consolidation
Lung disease

Perfusion:
PE
Hypovolaemia

$$DO_2 = CO \times Hb \times SaO_2 \times 1.34$$

SV x HR —— Slow Irregular Fast

Preload (CVP)
Contractility
Afterload (SVR)

21
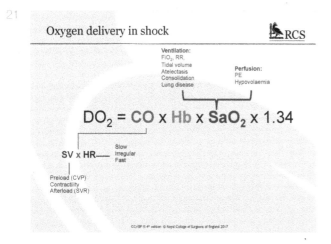

Oxygen delivery in shock

Ventilation:
FiO$_2$, RR,
Tidal volume
Atelectasis
Consolidation
Lung disease

Perfusion:
PE
Hypovolaemia

$$DO_2 = CO \times Hb \times SaO_2 \times 1.34$$

SV x HR —— Slow Irregular Fast

Preload (CVP)
Contractility
Afterload (SVR)

22
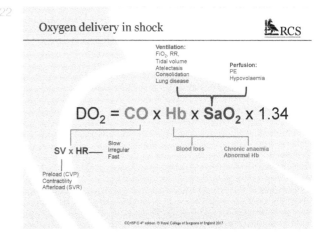

Oxygen delivery in shock

Ventilation:
FiO$_2$, RR,
Tidal volume
Atelectasis
Consolidation
Lung disease

Perfusion:
PE
Hypovolaemia

$$DO_2 = CO \times Hb \times SaO_2 \times 1.34$$

SV x HR —— Slow Irregular Fast

Preload (CVP)
Contractility
Afterload (SVR)

Blood loss   Chronic anaemia
               Abnormal Hb

23
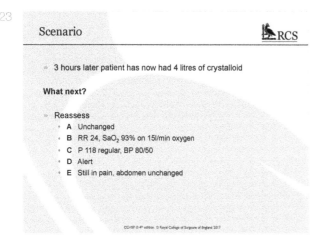

Scenario

- 3 hours later patient has now had 4 litres of crystalloid

What next?

- Reassess
  - A Unchanged
  - B RR 24, SaO$_2$ 93% on 15l/min oxygen
  - C P 118 regular, BP 80/50
  - D Alert
  - E Still in pain, abdomen unchanged

24
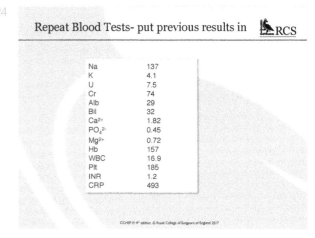

Repeat Blood Tests- put previous results in

Na	137
K	4.1
U	7.5
Cr	74
Alb	29
Bil	32
Ca^{2+}	1.82
PO$_4^{2-}$	0.45
Mg^{2+}	0.72
Hb	157
WBC	16.9
Plt	185
INR	1.2
CRP	493

ABG on 15 l/min O₂

pH	7.46
PaCO₂	3.9 kPa
PaO₂	12.0 kPa
HCO₃⁻	20.7 mmol/l
BE	-1.5 mmol/l
Lactate	2.9 mmol/l
Glucose 9.6 mmol/l	

Summarise the situation now

- Patient has had resuscitation with oxygen and fluids and is still tachycardic and hypotensive with a high lactate.
- Plan
  - Ask critical care for advice and assistance

What can Critical Care do to assist?

- Maximise supportive therapy
  - Optimise ventilation
  - (Invasive) cardiovascular monitoring
  - Cardiovascular manipulation
  - Other organ system monitoring
  - Co-ordination of care e.g. optimise analgesia

How critical care uses additional monitoring:

- Is all the oxygen delivered to the tissues used for metabolism?
- Oxygen extraction ratios
  - Can't be directly manipulated but
  - can be used to monitor adequacy of therapy e.g. severe sepsis.
  - Measure central venous oxygen saturations

Oxy-Haemoglobin Dissociation Curve

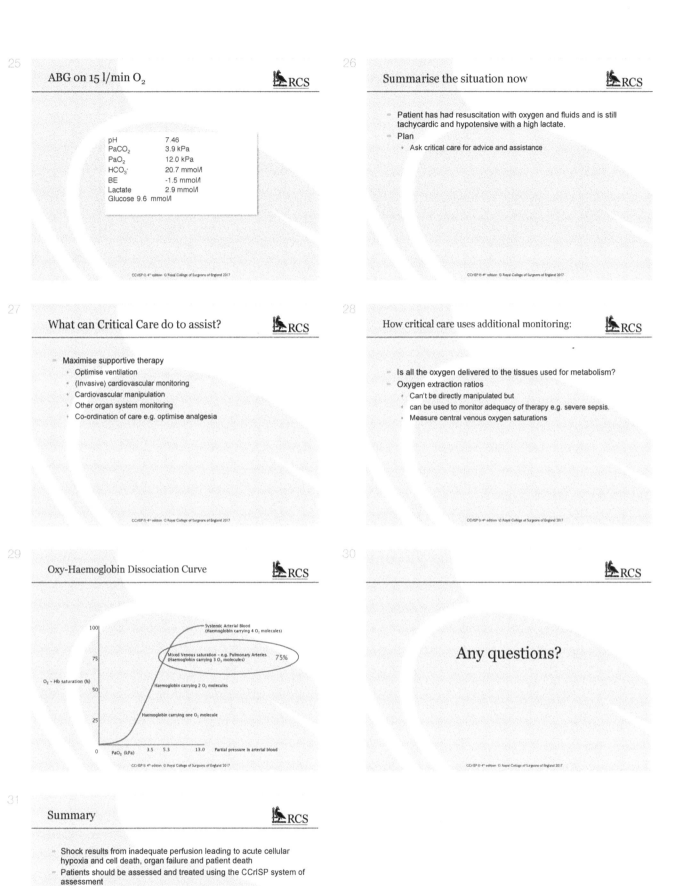

Any questions?

Summary

- Shock results from inadequate perfusion leading to acute cellular hypoxia and cell death, organ failure and patient death
- Patients should be assessed and treated using the CCrISP system of assessment
- Understanding the linkage between the physiological variables enables correct additional treatments to be started to optimise oxygen delivery

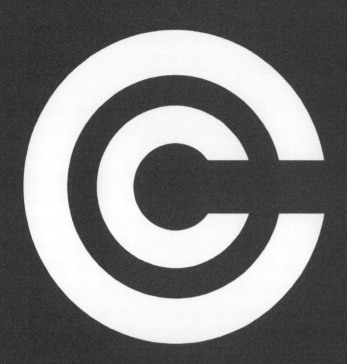

1.13

Small group session
Professional skills

Introduction

This is the first of two small group sessions focusing on professional, communication and decision-making skills. During this session the candidates will practise communication and organisational skills central to their developing role within the surgical team. Surgical trainees are often unaware of how important these skills are in successful practice.

Duration	45 minutes for each session (parts 1 and 2)
Style	Practical rotation (four groups of four candidates)
Faculty	One or two, plus an actor
AV	None

Learning outcomes

At the end of this session, participants will be able to:

- demonstrate the range of communication skills needed in surgical critical care;

- model some of these through clinical scenarios;

- formulate constructive feedback to peers.

Teaching outline

The professional skills small group session involves four scenarios. Each candidate must complete one scenario during the session. It is worth emphasising to the candidates that they will learn as much from watching and thinking about their colleagues' approaches as they do from practising the scenarios themselves.

Each block of four scenarios should take 45 minutes, and the whole block is repeated for each new group. It is important to maintain the pace and direction of this part of the programme, as this makes it more attractive and interesting for those taking part. For each scenario, there are topics and objectives, a brief for the participant and information for the actor and/or faculty. The instructor reads the participant brief out to the remainder of the group.

These scenarios are intended to be based on realistic situations and to cover a range of basic communication skills. A semi-structured approach has been developed in which scenarios are prepared in advance and this material is then used during the sessions, with an actor contributing an active role.

The session is introduced with routine introductions of presenters and format.

After each scenario, ask for reflections from the other participants and to briefly sum up the points covered. This style is used to try to encourage reflection, to highlight good aspects of communication and to identify any problems. At the end of each scenario, and at the end of each set of scenarios, the person leading should emphasise successes achieved and points covered.

It is important that candidates do not lose confidence in their abilities while at the same time realising that there is scope for some improvement.

Some faculty members use a whiteboard or flipchart to show three or four brief bullet points that summarise the scenario while it is in progress. The board can also be used to note down the topics covered by the scenario as they are discussed. These can then be used in the summary.

Timeline

Good timekeeping is vital. All four scenarios should be reviewed in the session and the actor fully briefed by the faculty involved before the session starts.

Introduction	2 minutes
Scenario 1	10 minutes*
Scenario 2	10 minutes*
Scenario 3	10 minutes*
Scenario 4	10 minutes*
Questions and summary	3 minutes

Leave time to take questions, summarise and close at the end.

*Allow at least 3 minutes for critiquing discussion and feedback.

Resources

▶ Briefs for participants/notes for instructors. p. 91–97

▶ Flipchart or white board and pens (for objectives and points).

▶ An actor.

▶ Scenario 1 (p. 93).

▶ Scenario 2 (p. 94).

▶ Scenario 3 (p. 95).

▶ Scenario 4 (p. 97).

Overview of all scenarios

The students will observe and discuss the following communication episodes.

Amputation

Demonstrate empathy, rapport and effective communication with a patient.

Informing a patient of ureteric injury

Demonstrate effective communication, in particular explain future complications and accept responsibility.

Explaining an emergency operation to a relative

Demonstrate an understanding of the nature of consent and assent in emergency treatment, avoid jargon and break bad news demonstrating skills of checking back and explaining.

Explaining futility of emergency surgery to a relative

Demonstrate sensitive handling of bad news, effective communication, empathy and active listening when talking to a relative.

Scenario 1: Amputation

Topics/objectives

- To explore issues pertaining to 'difficult' or 'hostile' patients.

- To understand the importance of empathy, honesty, rapport and effective communication in all patient interactions.

Brief for participant

During your duty weekend, a patient admitted under your team's care on Thursday comes to require an above-knee amputation. The patient, a 73-year-old widower, was admitted with pedal gangrene and rest pain following a long period of claudication. This had not been diagnosed in the community and, on admission, diabetes was also discovered. The limb is non-salvageable and amputation is needed before life or renal function is threatened directly.

The patient is not happy and you have been called to discuss matters further and obtain consent for surgery.

Brief for actor

The patient had complained to his GP about his claudication but no diagnosis or referral seems to have been made. The patient lost his wife to metastatic pancreatic cancer 2 years ago – in his eyes also diagnosed at a late stage. Complaints made about the care his wife received were not supported by the local authorities. He has lost faith in the medical profession, in the ability of medical practitioners to diagnose or treat, and suspects that they also cover up for each other. He is worried how he will cope with life in his two-storey house with one leg and wonders how he will make it to the bathroom (upstairs) in time. He has no close family nearby. He has not established much rapport with the nursing staff and is expressing doubts about whether he should have the operation.

The participant should try and understand your fears and concerns and acknowledge that all may not have been well in the past. They should empathise with you, try and establish rapport and communicate the current problem and its urgency in simple clear terms. The participant should not lie about the risks of intervention or about the struggles that amputees can face.

Discuss

This is someone who has lost faith in the medical profession and requires considerable reassurance and empathy. However, he must not be offered false hope simply to make the communication episode easier for the participant. While every effort will be made to try to ensure that the patient will walk with a prosthesis and 'get back to normal', the reality is that a reasonable proportion of such patients will achieve a lower level of independence following an amputation of this sort.

Scenario 2: Informing a patient of ureteric injury

Explaining a surgical error to patient. Information for participants.

Topics/objectives

- Communication.

- Explanation of potential future complications.

- Accepting responsibility.

Brief for participant

During a right hemicolectomy for a mobile caecal cancer on Mr Brown, you inadvertently divide the right ureter. You recognise the error at the time and call your consultant, who, along with the on-call urology consultant, reimplants the ureter and inserts a ureteric stent. It is the following morning on the ward round and the patient has not yet been told about the ureteric injury.

You are conducting the ward round. You assess the patient, who is doing well postoperatively, and asks how the operation went. He is concerned because he has noticed that the urine draining in his catheter bag is blood stained, and has been asking to see a doctor.

You need to inform the patient of the damage to the ureter.

Brief for actor

An actor should play the role of the patient. He should express concern about the blood in his urine. If the candidate fails to aknowledge that a mistake has been made or fails to empathise or reassure, the actor can become angry.

Brief for faculty

The candidate should be able to explain clearly what has happened, accept responsibility for it, and discuss possible longer term implications. If there are factual gaps in the candidate's knowledge it would be reasonable for them to suggest getting advice from senior or urological colleagues.

Scenario 3: Explain emergency operation to relative

Scenarios 3 and 4 relate to essentially the same case history but affect patients of very different age and fitness. The brief is written for an actor in middle age but could be adapted quite easily.

Topics/objectives

- To demonstrate understanding of the difference between consent and assent in emergency treatment.

- To communicate avoiding use of jargon.

- To demonstrate an empathetic approach to breaking bad news.

- To demonstrate ability to confirm understanding by use of checking back and explanation.

Brief for participant

A 63-year-old, previously fit, man presents with a 3-day history of lower abdominal pain. It worsened suddenly about 4 hours ago and he came to the emergency department. He is clearly shocked with peritonitis and is being resuscitated as plans are made for a prompt laparotomy. He is systemically ill with hypoxia, hypotension and oliguria. You have judged him to lack capacity and is unable to sign his own consent form. His partner has arrived and the nurse asks you, the surgical registrar, to speak to her before you go to the operating room to carry out what you expect will most likely be a Hartmann's procedure for sigmoid perforation.

Brief for actor

The actor should play the part of the wife (or another relative if this is more appropriate). She should ask questions about the degree of risk and any complications and should be prepared to follow these questions through if evasive answers are given ('Could it be cancer? He isn't going to die, is he?'). Similarly, if frightening answers are given, then these too should be pursued. The wife should be naturally distressed about her husband's condition and may sometimes not take things in as a consequence. She should also ask, if appropriate, if the surgeon is requesting consent for this procedure. The operation will probably result in a colostomy, which in many cases is not later reversed.

Discuss

This is a common task for the surgeon on call. It combines several complex communication skills. There is the need to explain the procedure without the use of medical jargon – in other words, it should be to do with making effective communication and explanation. However, in the background, there is also an element of breaking bad news and a distressed relative. These matters also need to be taken into account and a skill that might be helpful is that of checking back. Does the candidate check that the partner has really understood what has been said? The candidate should have some information to hand about the degree of risk involved and the likely side-effects and should be prepared to share this – the words 'death', 'colostomy' and 'cancer' should all usually feature. The candidate should also realise that the relative cannot be asked for consent.

Additional faculty information

In this case a laparotomy is appropriate, and in the patient's best interests. However, in the case of a patient whose capacity is impaired, the Mental Capacity Act states that the following should be borne in mind:

- past wishes of the patient

- religious beliefs

- views of relevant others (spouse).

The patient lacks the capacity to consent, although this loss is temporary. It is worth discussing how to assess capacity, ie to have capacity to make a decision a person should be able to:

- understand the information;

- retain that information;

- use or weigh up that information;

- communicate his or her decision

Discussion of capacity is also covered session 2.1, Ward dilemmas.

Scenario 4: Explaining the futility of emergency surgery to a relative

Topics covered

- An approach to handling 'bad news' conversations.

- Effective communication.

- Skills of empathy.

Brief for participant

An 87-year-old man is admitted from a care home with a probable 3-day history of steadily worsening lower abdominal pain. Despite 3 hours of intensive resuscitative treatment, he remains profoundly shocked with peritonitis, hypoxia, hypotension and oligo-anuria. The home carer has indicated that the patient never goes out and needs help with feeding, dressing and toileting on account of two previous cerebrovascular accidents and chronic respiratory disease. His daughter has arrived and the nurse asks you, the registrar, to speak to her. The daughter is asking if he is going to have an operation for the peritonitis.

Brief for actor/faculty

The actor should be briefed to be moderately distressed. If the candidate copes reasonably, the actor should question the decision not to operate but allow herself to be persuaded by appropriate explanation. If not, the candidate may ask the consultant to come in and carry out a procedure or assess the patient personally. Some candidates will not have clarified their objective and can get lost early in the scenario, failing to achieve the objective required for this patient. The instructors have the option, should the initial consultation go badly, of introducing a second part to the scenario involving a telephone call to the consultant responsible for the patient.

Discuss

In this case, it is not appropriate to subject the patient to surgery as the prospects of survival to hospital discharge are virtually nil. The patient would almost certainly need intensive care after surgery and the burden of organ supports would be great with no realistic prospect of survival. It is appropriate and humane to treat the patient conservatively.

The objective is to be able to handle a realistic discussion about the prognosis of surgery and reasons. Often family members are more realistic than doctors about the ability of their aged relatives to withstand surgery. There is potentially a lot of emotional distress and the candidate should demonstrate effective communication and empathy.

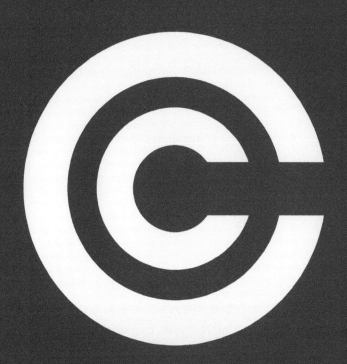

Small group session
Acute kidney injury

Participants revise the basics of renal function, and define acute kidney injury (AKI). Case scenarios then explore candidates' understanding of the basic management principles of acute kidney injury in surgical care.

Duration	45 min
Style	Scenario-based group discussion
Faculty	One or two
AV	PowerPoint presentation

Materials

▶ 1.14.0 Aute Kidney Injury Network (AKIN) classification and normal laboratory values.

Learning outcomes

At the end of this session, participants will be able to:

- summarise the functions of the kidney;

- summarise ways of measuring renal function;

- explain the rationale for and use of the AKIN classification to recognise acute kidney injury;

- outline the management of AKI in the surgical patient using the framework advocated by the CCrISP course;

- outline a simple plan for managing elective surgery in patients with chronic kidney disease.

Recommended timeline

Introduction   5 minutes (**slides 1–6**)

Scenarios   35 minutes
You are advised to cover at least three scenarios and always
include scenario 5, which deals with chronic kidney disease (see
'Notes on the scenarios', p. 98)

Questions/summary   5 minutes (maximum)

Teaching outline (slides 1–6)

Slides 1–6 form the introduction to the session, set objectives and provide a synopsis of renal function emphasising the AKIN criteria. **Slide 6** should be used to emphasise that the CCrISP assessment algorithm is to be used in dealing with patients of concern, as it will help to delineate and manage the underlying problems irrespective of cause.

Notes on introductory slides

The slides are should be revision of candidates' existing knowledge. The instructor can discuss factors that predispose to acute kidney injury and the pathophysiology of acute kidney injury in terms of aetiology, progress and recovery, information that is included in pre-course learning materials.

Other points to note when considering delivering this session:

- If discussing measures of renal function, instructors should emphasise the importance of urine output and baseline blood tests in the acutely ill patient. Other tests [estimated glomerular filtration rate (eGFR), fractional excretion of sodium, etc] can accurately reflect renal function but are not necessarily rapidly obtainable in an emergency, and in acute settings can change dramatically over a period of a few hours.

- Note that some of the scenarios contain a reference to eGFR, as this is routinely calculated and reported in some hospitals, but it does not form the basis of any of the internationally accepted definitions of AKI.

- AKI definitions (**slide 5**) have been developed over the last 10–12 years (previous criteria known as RIFLE criteria) and reflect the fact that urine output and serum creatinine are the two measures of renal function that are least influenced by non-renal pathologies.

- Predisposing factors can be discussed within each scenario.

- Traditional generic classifications of AKI emphasising *pre-renal* (usually hypoperfusion in hypovolaemic or septic states), *intrinsic damage* and *post-renal* or *obstructive* aetiologies can also be discussed, but the priority remains discussion about clinical management.

- Further points to consider as the skill station progresses:

  - The injured kidney (while not the cause of critical illness) can subsequently exaggerate and drive the inflammatory process.

  - Despite abnormal renal function, cell death (necrosis or apoptosis) does not necessarily occur, ie critical illness may lead to cells entering a form of 'suspended animation' or so-called **aestivation**, possibly explaining both normal post-mortem renal biopsies and relatively rapid recovery of renal function in many survivors of multiorgan dysfunction syndrome.

Notes on the scenarios

All scenarios are independent of each other. Explanations are available for instructors. A **minimum of three** scenarios should be covered and should include scenario 5 as a means of emphasising the implications of chronic kidney disease in patients presenting for surgery (elective or emergency). The cases illustrate many points of relevance for good general surgical care, so highlight these as well as those related directly to renal dysfunction. Scenario 1 is usually a good starting point. Allow the candidates to work through it and develop an understanding as to how the station runs.

Keep the session interactive, involving all candidates, and where possible attempt to place them in hypothetical situations of seniority when discussing the cases as a means of developing and assessing their professional and leadership skills. There are many other opportunities to pose questions around these cases, creating potential for it to become one of the most productive sections of the course. Leave time a maximum of 5 minutes to take questions, summarise and close.

Scenario 1 (slides 7–13)

In this case, patient management has been suboptimal, leading to AKI. It can be used to allow candidates to identify the points at which patient care could have been improved and they could have intervened. Questions to be considered appear on the slides.

A 65-year-old woman is admitted to the surgical ward with a history of sudden-onset (5 hours) severe pain and loss of function in both legs.

She is known to have a prosthetic aortic valve and atrial fibrillation. She takes digoxin, diuretics and warfarin.

Examination

A Airway patent.

B RR 20.

C HR 110 bpm, BP 120/75 mmHg, CRT 4 seconds.

D Alert, pupils normal, BM 6 mmol/L.

E Lower limbs pale, paraesthetic and pulseless.

Blood results

Na^+	134 mmol/L
K^+	4.7 mmol/L
Creatinine	178 µmol/L
Urea	10.5 mmol
eGFR	35 mL/min/1.73 m²
Venous bicarbonate	19 mmol/L
Albumin	36 g/L

Chest X-ray

This shows cardiomegaly, no oedema and the presence of a Starr–Edwards prosthesis.

Initial management

The initial management is radiological demonstration of saddle embolus followed by Fogarty embolectomy and removal of as much distal thrombus as possible. Poor perfusion beyond the popliteal artery on the right persists. Continue intra-arterial thrombolytic infusion (altepase).

Day 1

There is considerable haemorrhage around the femoral puncture site. The patient has experienced episodes of hypotension overnight.

Oliguria is present (250 mL in 12 hours). Blood on Stix test: ++++.

A diuretic has been given, with some effect: 250 mL over 4 hours, then 15 mL/h.

Day 2

Repeat CT angiography shows resolution of thrombus. The patient remains oliguric and short of breath. The left lower leg is painful and tense on dorsiflexion of foot.

Na^+	143 mmol/L
K^+	4.1 mmol/L
Creatinine	291 μmol/L
Urea	21.6 mmol/L
eGFR	15 mL/min/1.73 m^2
HCO_3^-	14 mmol/L
Albumin	18 g/L
Ca^{2+}	1.69 mmol/L
PO_4^{3-}	2.38 mmol/L
CPK	34 000 IU/L
Platelets	84×10^9/L
Hb	85 g/L

Background information and discussion points for the instructor

Adequacy of overnight management of the patient and contribution of pathologies towards AKI:

- Management plan unclear (including management of coagulation status).
- Dilemma of balancing anticoagulant therapies.
- Hypotension, haemorrhage and oliguria not effectively dealt with.

Consequences of prolonged ischaemia of legs:

- Significant muscle injury leading to compartment syndrome is highly likely.

- Potential for hypovolaemia secondary to considerable extracellular fluid (ECF) loss into damaged tissue.

- Products of muscle injury (note raised phosphate and CPK) likely to cause renal tubular injury.

Prevention/reduction of severity

- Maintenance of adequate circulating volume.

- The use of diuretics as the first-line response to oliguria is not acceptable.

Should revascularisation of the right leg have been attempted at presentation?

Would prophylactic fasciotomies or possibly compartment pressure monitoring have been indicated?

The nephrotoxic effects of radio-opaque dye in the hypovolaemic patient should be stressed.

Ca^{2+} is low as a result of calcium binding to dead muscle and low albumin.

The low HCO_3^- reflects buffering as the response to the metabolic acidaemia.

The low albumin is a consequence of capillary leak and redistribution of albumin in response to inflammation from muscle injury and reperfusion of the leg.

The patient should be aggressively resuscitated and referred to critical care, where cardiovascular optimisation should be considered, prior to fasciotomy.

Beware of the potential life-threatening potassium rise after fasciotomy in conjunction with acute renal failure. Discussion about the management of hyperkalaemia can occur at this point (note that the patient in scenario 3 has hyperkalaemia).

Reassessment and amputation may be needed as an immediately life-saving intervention.

Slide 14 provides a summary of some of these points.

Scenario 2 (slides 15–20)

A 64-year-old woman with known ischaemic heart disease has been admitted with a 48-hour history of abdominal pain and vomiting. By the evening the pain had moved to the right iliac fossa, frank peritonism was present and a laparotomy was performed.

At induction of anaesthesia she was given prophylactic antibiotics and at operation she was found to have faecal peritonitis and a perforated inflammatory mass in the region of her caecum/ascending colon. She underwent a hemicolectomy, ileostomy and mucous fistula. On opening the abdomen and after initial manipulation of the bowel she suffered severe hypotension.

At 10pm in the recovery area she remained intubated and ventilated awaiting a critical care bed with an arterial line and right internal jugular central line in place. The core trainee in anaesthesia is considering extubation and a recent set of observations and blood results are shown below.

HR	105 bpm
CRT	3 seconds
BP	160/100 mmHg
CVP	7 mmHg, peripherally shut down
Temperature	35.3°C
PO_2	20 kPa (150 mmHg) (FiO_2 0.6)
PCO_2	5.7 kPa (41.8 mmHg)
pH	7.29
HCO_3^-	19 mmol/L
BE	−4.8 mmol/L
Hb	128 g/L
Na^+	152 mmol/L
WBC	2.2×10^9/L
K^+	3.7 mmol/L
Platelets	189×10^9/L
PT	21 seconds (13 seconds)
Creatinine	112 µmol/L
APPT	65 seconds (46 seconds)
Urea	13 mmol/L

- Should the patient be extubated?

- Justify your reasoning.

Six hours postoperatively (slide 18)

After active warming, the patient is vasodilated, tachycardic, hypotensive and oliguric and serum creatinine is increasing.

- What would you do?

- What are your concerns?

Candidates should suggest further fluid boluses and resuscitation at this point with a possible need for vasopressors.

The patient is now on pressors.

- Is the patient stable? (No)

- Has she suffered an AKI? (Yes)

- Is renal replacement therapy (RRT) indicated? (Not at this point. Reassess and optimise with further fluid if possible. RRT may be needed later.)

Discussion points

There is evidence of multiorgan dysfunction (as shown by a requirement for invasive ventilation and relative hypoxaemia, intraoperative hypotension, coagulopathy, metabolic acidaemia and hypothermia). It would be unwise to extubate the patient until she has stabilised further in a critical care facility and has rewarmed (**slides 16** and **17**).

The patient's circulation will need to be managed carefully, as the development of severe peripheral vasodilatation and increased vascular permeability is likely. This process is potentially beginning to occur (**slide 18**) and the failure of response to fluid challenges with a rise in creatinine to 204 µmol/L should be noted by the candidates (**slide 19**). Likely aetiologies are vasodilatation as a result of severe sepsis/sepsis syndrome, and hypovolaemia due to the loss of intravascular and interstitial fluid into the peritoneal space as part of the on-going inflammatory process is also relevant.

Low diastolic pressures can impair coronary artery blood flow (the left coronary artery being particularly dependent on diastolic pressures for flow), a situation further compounded by a tachycardia (shortening diastole), leaving the patient (who is known to have ischaemic heart disease) at increased risk of an acute coronary event.

Invasive cardiovascular monitoring is already established and measurement of cardiac output is recommended to optimise the cardiovascular status with either vasoconstrictors and/or inotropes (this makes the link to other sections of the course).

After 36 hours the patient has been stabilised, but needs high levels of support (**slide 19**). The supported cardiovascular status appears to be close to optimal but she remains oliguric and has suffered an AKI, as shown by a 1.8-fold increase in serum creatinine. Further fluid challenges at this point would be reasonable but are unlikely to produce a dramatic improvement. There is no rule about when to commence RRT, but a discussion about the indications for RRT (**slide 20**) is warranted in this case and, unless there were definitive signs pointing towards the futility of RRT, it should be given strong consideration in this case.

Scenario 3 (slides 21–23)

A 51-year-old woman is admitted to the urology ward with vomiting, anorexia and postural dizziness. She also complains of shortness of breath, which has been getting worse over the past 2 weeks.

She has had her right kidney removed in the past (baseline creatinine is 143 μmol/L), as it had been destroyed by chronic pyelonephritis. She has subsequently been troubled with recurrent ureteric colic in her left kidney.

She has a NEWS of 7 on initial assessment:

RR	25/min	Score = 3
SaO$_2$	100% (air)	Score = 0
Temperature	37.7°C	Score = 0
BP	94/45 mmHg	Score = 2
HR	123 bpm, sinus rhythm	Score = 2
AVPU	Alert	Score = 0

Arterial blood gas and biochemistry (slide 21)

pH	7.25
PO$_2$	110 mmHg (14.6 kPa) (FiO$_2$ 0.21)
PCO$_2$	24 mmHg (3.2 kPa)
HCO$_3^-$	11 mmol
BE	−9.1 mmol/L
Lactate	2.4 mmol
Na$^+$	135 mmol/L
K$^+$	5.9 mmol/L
Urea	26 mmol/L
Creatinine	369 μmol/L
CXR	NAD

10 mL urine when catheterised

- What is developing?

- How should the problem be corrected?

▢ Acute kidney injury (2.6-fold increase in serum creatinine, albeit over an indeterminate time interval) secondary to obstruction.

▢ Remember to exclude obstruction in any case of renal failure.

▢ An appropriate assessment and plan is therefore required (CCrISP algorithm will structure the response and plan to the NEWS alert):

National Early Warning Score	Minimum frequency of monitoring	Clinical response
0	12-hourly observations	Continue routine NEWS monitoring with every set of observations
Total: 1–4	4-hourly observations	Inform registered nurse, who must assess the patient
		Registered nurse to decide if increased frequency of monitoring and/or escalation of critical care is required
Total: 5 or more or 3 in one parameters	Hourly observations	NEWS responder
		Response time 30 minutes
Total; 7 or more or 3 in two parameters	Continuous observations	Senior NEWS responder **and** outreach
		Response time 10 minutes

Stop. Think. Why has my patient triggered?

Treat hyperkalaemia (see below) and relieve the obstruction by appropriate surgical or radiological means (percutaneous/extracorporeal/surgical) depending on the cause. Antegrade nephrostomy may also be required.

Management of hyperkalaemia

▢ Stop any potassium.

▢ Treat the cause.

▢ Give calcium resonium (ion exchange).

▢ Administer dextrose/insulin (promotes intracellular uptake of potassium).

▢ Administer salbutamol. (Acts by inducing hyperglycaemia, increasing production of endogenous insulin and subsequent intracellular uptake of potassium).

▢ Administer calcium chloride/calcium gluconate (provides myocardial protection from the hyperkalaemia).

- Administer bicarbonate (increases pH and exchange of potassium and hydrogen ions).

- Institute renal replacement therapy (haemofiltration, haemodialysis).

The patient can be made more or less septic as you wish (note that there is a whole session on 'unwell surgical patients' so do not get sidetracked). Discuss the importance of the combination of obstruction and infection – rapid renal destruction, severe sepsis.

Scenario 4 (slides 24–26)

A 65-year-old female patient (48 kg and 1.60 m; BMI 18.7) with moderately severe renal dysfunction due to diabetic nephropathy (baseline creatinine 239 µmol/L) has undergone a total hip replacement for osteoarthritis. She has been prescribed morphine PCA with 'standard settings' for postoperative analgesia, ie 1 mg bolus, 5-minute lock-out, zero background infusion and no 4-hourly limit.

She has a NEWS of 7 on initial assessment:

RR	11/min	Score = 1
SaO$_2$	98% (4 L/min)	Score = 2
Temperature	36.9°C	Score = 0
BP	104/56 mmHg	Score = 1
HR	85/min, regular	Score = 0
AVPU	P	Score = 3

Further neurological assessment (if candidates ask):

- opens eyes to pain

- localises to pain

- incomprehensible sounds

- Glasgow Coma Scale score = 8

- pupils 2 mm bilaterally with minimal reactivity.

Biochemistry

Na+	131 mmol/L
K+	4.5 mmol/L
Creatinine	225 µmol/L

Arterial blood gases

PO_2	68 mmHg (9.1 kPa) (FiO_2 0.3)
PCO_2	78 mmHg (10.4 kPa)
pH	7.18
Bicarbonate	23 mmol
BE	–2.5 mmol/L

- What has happened?

- What should be done now?

- How might this have been prevented?

Discussion points (slide 26)

Morphine metabolites have been retained and accumulated as a result of the renal compromise and the patient now has CO_2 narcosis. The patient is also small and the 'standard' setting of the morphine dose may have been relatively high for her.

The opiate should be reversed and careful observations begun. A small dose of naloxone may suffice and possibly minimise difficulties with severe pain and distress that can occur if an excessive dose of naloxone is given as a bolus. Doses of naloxone often need to be repeated and candidates should be aware of this, plus the potential to observe the patient in a different setting, ie critical care. There is the chance to link to Pain Management (session 2.2) and emphasise the need for consideration of alternative methods of analgesia.

Recognise this risk in patients with renal compromise – **predict and prevent**!

Scenario 5 (slides 27–30)

A 69-year-old man with end-stage renal disease (ESRD) and diabetes is an elective admission for repair of an incisional hernia. He has hypertension and ischaemic heart disease.

He underwent a laparotomy 2 years previously for peritonitis and removal of an infected peritoneal dialysis catheter. Since then he has undergone intermittent haemodialysis three times a week. Despite this he has a functional status of 6.9 METs.

Medical history

- Type II diabetes mellitus including diabetic nephropathy resulting in ESRD (managed with oral hypoglycaemic agents).

- Hypertension.

- Ischaemic heart disease and an ECG showing sinus rhythm and a Q-wave in aVF (possibly indicating an old inferior myocardial infarction).

- CXR: NAD.

- Functional status: 6.9 METs (this equates to climbing two flights of stairs, so is reasonable considering his comorbidities)

Blood results (slide 28)

Hb	108 g/L
WCC	6.7×10^9/L
Pl	260×10^9/L
Na^+	138 mmol/L
K^+	5.3 mmol/L
Urea	36.1 mmol/L
Creatinine	498 µmol/L
Bilirubin	12 µmol/L
ALT	18 units/L
Alkaline phosphatase	54 units/L
PT	14 seconds
APPT	38 seconds
Glucose	7.5 mmol/L
HbA1c	4.5% (4–6%)
Arterial blood gases (air)	
pH	7.34
$PaCO_2$	4.6 kPa
PaO_2	10.3 kPa
HCO_3^-	21.3 mmol/L
BE	−4.6 mmol/L

The main considerations for perioperative management centre on an awareness of the pathophysiological consequences of ESRD (usually related to uraemia, eg poor wound healing, bleeding from platelet dysfunction), the effect of ESRD on drug function/drug interactions and the consequences of managing ESRD, eg the presence of arteriovenous fistula (AVF), dialysis catheters, etc.

As survival rates improve, more patients with ESRD are likely to present for elective surgery. As part of the background, the instructor may outline some issues about the relatively common presentation of patients with chronic kidney disease, eg there are in excess of 140,000 patients in the UK who have ESRD, of whom:

- approximately 37% are undergoing haemodialysis;

- 16–17% are receiving ambulatory peritoneal dialysis;

- the remainder have undergone renal transplantation (although this may be on the increase as live-related programmes expand).

Aetiologies include diabetes (30%), hypertension (24%), glomerulonephritis (17%) and multiple cases of unknown aetiology.

Slide 30

Other problems with patients with chronic renal failure or renal transplants coming to non-renal surgery include:

- cardiovascular comorbidities and other organs with chronic impairment

- anaemia

- uraemia and platelet dysfunction

- delayed gastric emptying

- poor tissue healing

- immunosuppression

- electrolyte abnormalities

- difficult intravascular access: AVF may limit sites and multiple line insertions make access difficult.

Slide 31 (questions)

Notes on the concluding section (slides 31 and 32)

Instructors should leave 5 minutes at the end for questions and the summary (**slide 32**) outlining the management of acute kidney injury and considerations for chronic kidney disease.

Appendix I: Acute Kidney Injury Network (AKIN) classification for acute renal failure

Acute Kidney Injury Network. Report of an initiative to improve outcomes in acute kidney injury. *Crit Care* 2007; **11**: R31–R38.

	GFR criteria	Urine output criteria
1	Increase in serum creatinine >26.4 µmol/L or 1.5–2.0× baseline	<0.5 mL/kg/h for more than 6 hours
2	Increase in serum creatine of 2–3× baseline	<0.5 mL/kg/h for more than 12 hours
3	Increase in creatine of ≥3× baseline or serum creatinine >354 µmol/L	<0.3 mL/kg/h for more than 24 hours
Loss	Persistent acute renal failure	
	Complete loss of kidney function for >4 weeks	
ESRD	End-stage renal disease (>3 months)	

Appendix 2: normal laboratory values

Measurement	Normal range
Sodium (Na⁺)	135–145 mmol/L
Potassium (K⁺)	3.5–5.0 mmol/L
Urea	3.1–7.9 mmol/L
Creatinine	
Male	64–104 µmol/L
Female	49–90 µmol/L
Total protein	58–78 g/L
Albumin	34–50 g/L
Calcium (Ca²⁺)	2.12–2.60 mmol/L
Phosphate (PO₄³⁻)	0.80–1.44 mmol/L
Bilirubin	0–19 µmol/L
Alkaline phosphatase (ALP)	35–120 units/L
Alanine aminotransferase (ALT)	0–45 units/L
Creatine kinase	
Male	38–174 units/L
Female	96–140 units/L
Haemoglobin (Hb)	130–180 g/L
Platelets	150–450 × 10⁹/L
White cell count (WCC)	4.0–11.0 × 10⁹/L
Prothrombin time (PT)	11.0–13.0 seconds
Activated partial thromboplastin time (APTT)	24–39 seconds
Fibrinogen	1.5–4.0 g/L
pH	7.35–7.45
$PaCO_2$	4.5–6.0 kPa (34–42 mmHg)
PaO_2	11.0–14.0 kPa (83–105 mmHg)
HCO_3^-	24–28 mmol/L
Base excess	–2 to +2 mmol/L
Lactate	0.4–1.7 mmol/L
Glucose	<11.1 mmol/L random
C-reactive protein (CRP)	0–5 mg/L
Chloride (Cl⁻)	95–108 mmol/L
Amylase	28–100 units/L

1

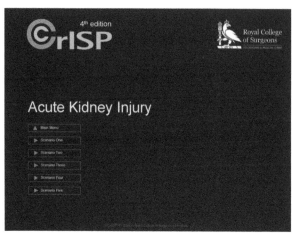

2

Learning Outcomes

- State the functions of the kidney
- Outline ways of measuring renal function
- Describe the rationale for and use of AKIN criteria in patients with AKI
- Specify the principles of management of AKI within the framework advocated by the CCrISP course

CCrISP® 4th Edition Royal College of Surgeons of England

3

What are the functions of the kidney?

- Fluid and electrolyte balance
- Acid-base balance
- Excretion of water soluble metabolites, toxins and drugs
- Endocrine:
  - Blood pressure control: renin and angiotensin
  - Vitamin D synthesis
  - Erythropoietin

CCrISP® 4th Edition Royal College of Surgeons of England

4

How can renal function be measured?

- Urine output
- Serum creatinine
- Serum urea
- Serum sodium and potassium
- Glomerular filtration rate (measured/estimated)
- Fractional excretion of sodium
- Urinary electrolytes

CCrISP® 4th Edition Royal College of Surgeons of England

5

Acute Kidney Injury (AKIN Criteria)

Stage	GFR criteria	Urine output criteria
1	Increase creat. >26.4µmol/l or 1.5 to 2.0 from baseline	<0.5ml/kg/hr over 6 hrs
2	Increase creat. x 2-3 from baseline	<0.5ml/kg/hr over 12 hrs
3	Increase creat. x 3 from baseline or serum creat > 354µmol/l	<0.3ml/kg/hr over 24 hrs

Loss	Persistent AKI. Complete loss of kidney function for > 4 wks
ESRD	End Stage Kidney Disease (> 3 months)

CCrISP® 4th Edition Royal College of Surgeons of England

6

The Management of Acute Kidney Injury

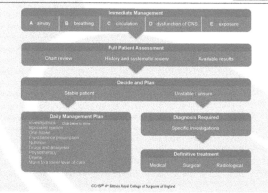

CCrISP® 4th Edition Royal College of Surgeons of England

7

Scenario One

- A 65-year-old woman is admitted to the surgical ward with a 5 hour history of sudden onset of severe pain and loss of function in both legs.
- She is known to have a prosthetic aortic valve and atrial fibrillation.
- She takes digoxin, diuretics and warfarin.

CCrISP® 4th Edition Royal College of Surgeons of England

8

Scenario One

- Airway patent
- RR 20 bpm
- HR 110 bpm, regular
- CRT 4 secs
  - Where? Fingers (yes) Toes? > 5 seconds
- BP: 120/75 mm/Hg
- Alert, pupils normal, BM 6mmol/l
- Lower limbs pale, paraesthetic and pulseless

What are the abnormalities and how would deal with them at this stage?

CCrISP® 4th Edition Royal College of Surgeons of England

9

Scenario One

- CXR cardiomegaly
  - no oedema
- Starr Edwards prosthesis

Na⁺	134 mmol/l
K⁺	4.7 mmol/l
Creat	178 μmol/l
Urea	10.5 mmol/l
eGFR	35
HCO₃	19 mmol/l
Albumin	36 g/l

What is your interpretation of the abnormalities?

What is your next step?

10

Scenario One: initial management

- CT angiogram: saddle embolus
- Management: embolectomy and removal of distal thrombus as possible
- Borderline poor perfusion beyond right popliteal artery
- Continuation of intra-arterial thrombolytic infusion (alteplase)

11

Scenario One: progress

- Day 1
  - Heparin infusion continued, wounds ooze +++
  - Episodes of hypotension overnight
  - Oliguria: 250 ml/12 hours
  - Haematuria: ++++ blood on stix test
  - Given diuretic resulting in increased urine output of 250 ml over 4 hours, then 15 ml/hour
- Day 2
  - Patient is SOB and is passing 15ml urine/hr for 6h
  - Foot well perfused, unaffected
  - CRT 3 seconds
  - Very tense calf, painful left lower leg on foot dorsiflexion

12

What is your working diagnosis?

- Compartment syndrome

13

Scenario One: progress

Na⁺	143 mmol/l
K⁺	4.1 mmol/l
Urea	21.6 mmol/l
Creat	291 μmol/l
eGFR	15 ml/min
HCO₃	14 mmol/l
Albumin	18 g/l
Ca²⁺	1.69 mmol/l
PO₄³⁻	2.38 mmol/l
CPK	34,000 IU/l
Hb	85 g/l
Platelets	84 x 10⁹/l
Lactate	3.4mmol/l

Could it have been prevented?

Why are the calcium and total HCO₃ low?

Why is the albumin low?

What should be done now?

14

Scenario One: points to consider

- Clear management plans are needed
- Prolonged leg ischaemia increases risks of AKI
- Role of fasciotomies/revascularisation
- Considerable biochemical disturbance
- Role of HCO₃ alkalinisation

15

Scenario Two

- A 64-year-old woman with known ischaemic heart disease is admitted with a 48 hour history of abdominal pain and vomiting.
- Within 4 hours:
  - Pain moved to the RIF
  - Peritonism (antibiotic therapy commenced)
  - Consent for surgery
- Laparotomy:
  - Faecal peritonitis: perforated inflammatory mass in region of caecum/ascending colon
  - BP (136/67 to 75/38 and 68/36 mm/Hg)
  - Hemi-colectomy, ileostomy and mucous fistula

16

Scenario Two: recovery area

- Ventilated, awaiting critical care bed
- Central line and arterial line in situ
- Observations
  - Temp: 35.3°C
  - HR: 105 bpm
  - BP: 160/100 mmHg
  - CVP: 7 mmHg
  - CRT: 3 secs

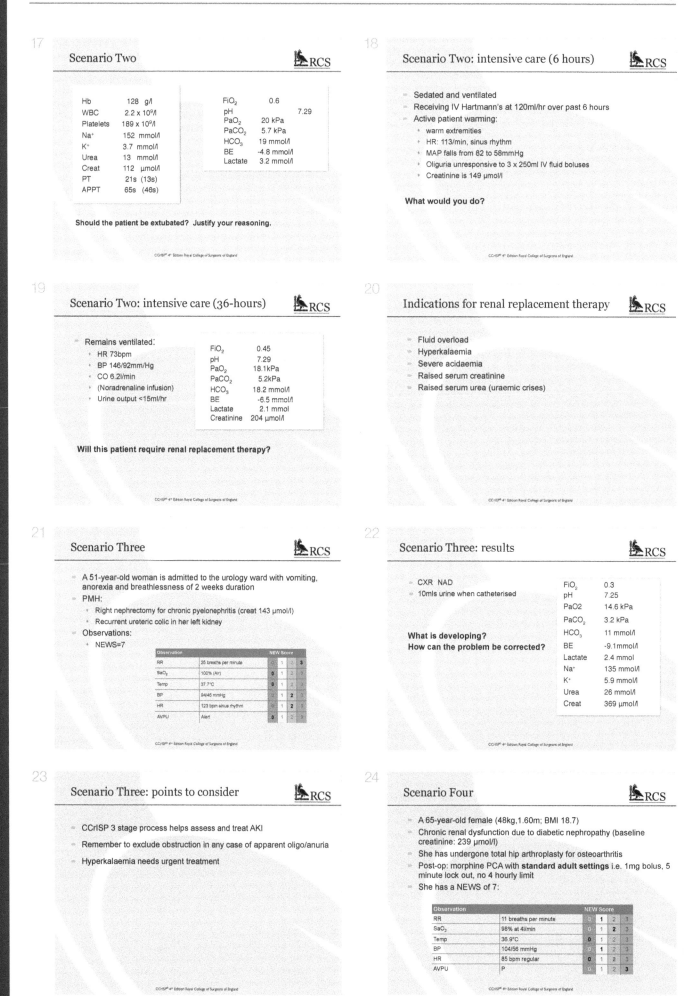

17

Scenario Two RCS

Hb	128 g/l	FiO₂	0.6	
WBC	2.2 x 10⁹/l	pH		7.29
Platelets	189 x 10⁹/l	PaO₂	20 kPa	
Na⁺	152 mmol/l	PaCO₂	5.7 kPa	
K⁺	3.7 mmol/l	HCO₃	19 mmol/l	
Urea	13 mmol/l	BE	-4.8 mmol/l	
Creat	112 μmol/l	Lactate	3.2 mmol/l	
PT	21s (13s)			
APPT	65s (46s)			

Should the patient be extubated? Justify your reasoning.

CCrISP® 4ᵗʰ Edition Royal College of Surgeons of England

18

Scenario Two: intensive care (6 hours) RCS

- Sedated and ventilated
- Receiving IV Hartmann's at 120ml/hr over past 6 hours
- Active patient warming:
  - warm extremities
  - HR: 113/min, sinus rhythm
  - MAP falls from 82 to 58mmHg
  - Oliguria unresponsive to 3 x 250ml IV fluid boluses
  - Creatinine is 149 μmol/l

What would you do?

CCrISP® 4ᵗʰ Edition Royal College of Surgeons of England

19

Scenario Two: intensive care (36-hours) RCS

- Remains ventilated:
  - HR 73bpm
  - BP 146/92mm/Hg
  - CO 6.2l/min
  - (Noradrenaline infusion)
  - Urine output <15ml/hr

FiO₂	0.45
pH	7.29
PaO₂	18.1kPa
PaCO₂	5.2kPa
HCO₃	18.2 mmol/l
BE	-6.5 mmol/l
Lactate	2.1 mmol
Creatinine	204 μmol/l

Will this patient require renal replacement therapy?

CCrISP® 4ᵗʰ Edition Royal College of Surgeons of England

20

Indications for renal replacement therapy RCS

- Fluid overload
- Hyperkalaemia
- Severe acidaemia
- Raised serum creatinine
- Raised serum urea (uraemic crises)

CCrISP® 4ᵗʰ Edition Royal College of Surgeons of England

21

Scenario Three RCS

- A 51-year-old woman is admitted to the urology ward with vomiting, anorexia and breathlessness of 2 weeks duration
- PMH:
  - Right nephrectomy for chronic pyelonephritis (creat 143 μmol/l)
  - Recurrent ureteric colic in her left kidney
- Observations:
  - NEWS=7

Observation		NEW Score			
RR	25 breaths per minute	0	1	2	**3**
SaO₂	100% (Air)	**0**	1	2	3
Temp	37.7°C	**0**	1	2	3
BP	94/45 mmHg	0	1	**2**	3
HR	123 bpm sinus rhythm	0	1	**2**	3
AVPU	Alert	**0**	1	2	3

CCrISP® 4ᵗʰ Edition Royal College of Surgeons of England

22

Scenario Three: results RCS

- CXR NAD
- 10mls urine when catheterised

What is developing?
How can the problem be corrected?

FiO₂	0.3
pH	7.25
PaO2	14.6 kPa
PaCO₂	3.2 kPa
HCO₃	11 mmol/l
BE	-9.1mmol/l
Lactate	2.4 mmol
Na⁺	135 mmol/l
K⁺	5.9 mmol/l
Urea	26 mmol/l
Creat	369 μmol/l

CCrISP® 4ᵗʰ Edition Royal College of Surgeons of England

23

Scenario Three: points to consider RCS

- CCrISP 3 stage process helps assess and treat AKI
- Remember to exclude obstruction in any case of apparent oligo/anuria
- Hyperkalaemia needs urgent treatment

CCrISP® 4ᵗʰ Edition Royal College of Surgeons of England

24

Scenario Four RCS

- A 65-year-old female (48kg, 1.60m; BMI 18.7)
- Chronic renal dysfunction due to diabetic nephropathy (baseline creatinine: 239 μmol/l)
- She has undergone total hip arthroplasty for osteoarthritis
- Post-op: morphine PCA with **standard adult settings** i.e. 1mg bolus, 5 minute lock out, no 4 hourly limit
- She has a NEWS of 7:

Observation		NEW Score			
RR	11 breaths per minute	0	**1**	2	3
SaO₂	98% at 4l/min	0	1	**2**	3
Temp	36.9°C	**0**	1	2	3
BP	104/56 mmHg	0	**1**	2	3
HR	85 bpm regular	**0**	1	2	3
AVPU	P	0	1	2	**3**

CCrISP® 4ᵗʰ Edition Royal College of Surgeons of England

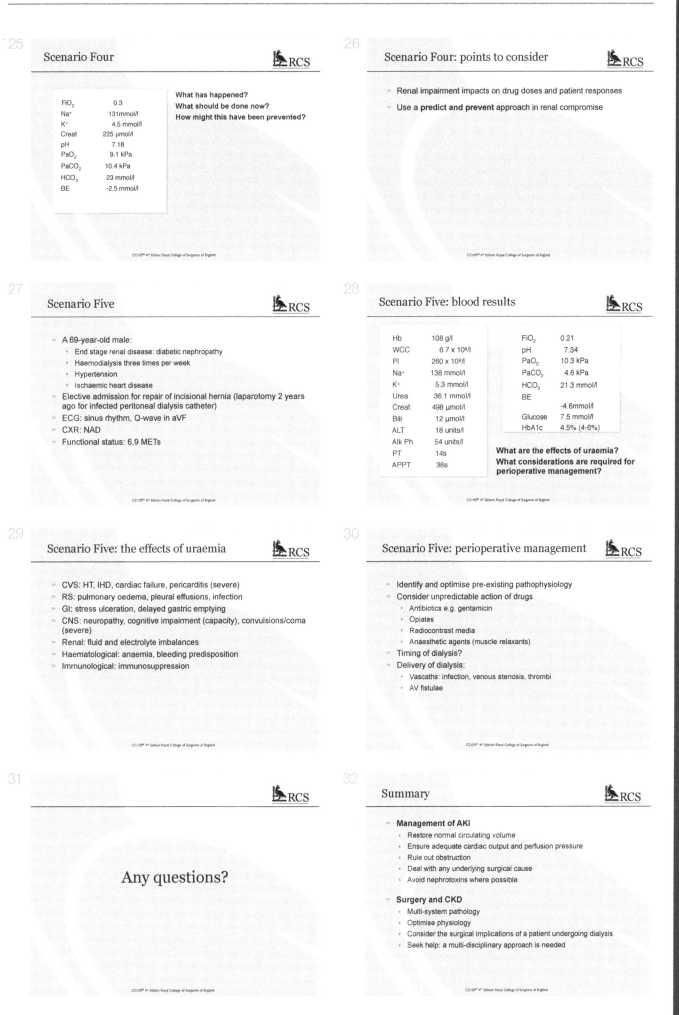

25

Scenario Four

FiO_2	0.3
Na^+	131mmol/l
K^+	4.5 mmol/l
Creat	225 µmol/l
pH	7.18
PaO_2	9.1 kPa
$PaCO_2$	10.4 kPa
HCO_3	23 mmol/l
BE	-2.5 mmol/l

What has happened?
What should be done now?
How might this have been prevented?

26

Scenario Four: points to consider

- Renal impairment impacts on drug doses and patient responses
- Use a **predict and prevent** approach in renal compromise

27

Scenario Five

- A 69-year-old male:
  - End stage renal disease: diabetic nephropathy
  - Haemodialysis three times per week
  - Hypertension
  - Ischaemic heart disease
- Elective admission for repair of incisional hernia (laparotomy 2 years ago for infected peritoneal dialysis catheter)
- ECG: sinus rhythm, Q-wave in aVF
- CXR: NAD
- Functional status: 6.9 METs

28

Scenario Five: blood results

Hb	108 g/l	FiO_2	0.21
WCC	6.7 x 10⁹/l	pH	7.34
Pl	260 x 10⁹/l	PaO_2	10.3 kPa
Na^+	138 mmol/l	$PaCO_2$	4.6 kPa
K^+	5.3 mmol/l	HCO_3	21.3 mmol/l
Urea	36.1 mmol/l	BE	
Creat	498 µmol/l		-4.6mmol/l
Bili	12 µmol/l	Glucose	7.5 mmol/l
ALT	18 units/l	HbA1c	4.5% (4-6%)
Alk Ph	54 units/l		
PT	14s		
APPT	38s		

What are the effects of uraemia?
What considerations are required for perioperative management?

29

Scenario Five: the effects of uraemia

- CVS: HT, IHD, cardiac failure, pericarditis (severe)
- RS: pulmonary oedema, pleural effusions, infection
- GI: stress ulceration, delayed gastric emptying
- CNS: neuropathy, cognitive impairment (capacity), convulsions/coma (severe)
- Renal: fluid and electrolyte imbalances
- Haematological: anaemia, bleeding predisposition
- Immunological: immunosuppression

30

Scenario Five: perioperative management

- Identify and optimise pre-existing pathophysiology
- Consider unpredictable action of drugs
  - Antibiotics e.g. gentamicin
  - Opiates
  - Radiocontrast media
  - Anaesthetic agents (muscle relaxants)
- Timing of dialysis?
- Delivery of dialysis:
  - Vascaths: infection, venous stenosis, thrombi
  - AV fistulae

31

Any questions?

32

Summary

- **Management of AKI**
  - Restore normal circulating volume
  - Ensure adequate cardiac output and perfusion pressure
  - Rule out obstruction
  - Deal with any underlying surgical cause
  - Avoid nephrotoxins where possible

- **Surgery and CKD**
  - Multi-system pathology
  - Optimise physiology
  - Consider the surgical implications of a patient undergoing dialysis
  - Seek help: a multi-disciplinary approach is needed

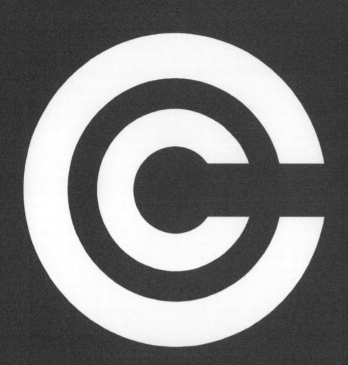

1.15

Group session
Nutrition

This session involves all 16 participants and is conducted as an interactive lecture. It is timetabled at the end of the first day and should allow one member of faculty to do this at the same time as the course director holds a faculty meeting. Case scenarios have been chosen to introduce consideration of enteral and parenteral nutrition from a theoretical and practical perspective and include a mixture of practical information and review of recent research evidence.

Duration	45 minutes
Style	Scenario-based group discussion
Faculty	One
AV	PowerPoint presentation

Learning outcomes

At the end of this session, participants will be able to:

- define the methods for providing nutritional support to patients;

- evaluate the benefits and risks of the different forms of nutritional support;

- characterise the role of the surgeon along with dietitians and nutrition teams in providing nutritional support;

- select appropriate forms of nutritional support for surgical patients.

Timeline

Introduction	1 minute (**slide 2**, learning outcomes)
Scenarios	40 minutes
Questions/summary	4 minutes

Teaching outline

Scenario 1 (slides 3–19)

This case deals with a young man caught in a house fire.

Although it would be expected that he could eat and drink, the case has been selected to illustrate the importance of checking the adequacy of nutritional intake using nutritional screening tools, the increased metabolic demands of acute illness and the role of nasogastric feeding in patients with an intact gastrointestinal tract.

Slides 6–9 illustrate the importance of nutritional assessment using the Malnutrition Universal Screening Tool (MUST) (**slide 7**), which has been chosen as it is the most widely used screening tool in the UK. **Slide 8** illustrates the ways in which erroneous estimates of nutritional status might be made, and **slide 9** makes the point that simple weight assessment can be deceptive.

Slides 13 and **14** should prompt discussion of the importance of ensuring correct nasogastric tube placement to prevent serious complications and risk of death if misplaced.

Slides 15–17 illustrate the evidence from the recent Calories trial, which compared enteral and parenteral feeding in critically ill patients. **Slide 16** shows data from the trial and can be omitted if necessary, as it is followed by a summary of results in **slide 17**. The trial showed no difference in the two methods and illustrates that ensuring adequacy of nutrition in critically ill patients is more important than the choice of route.

Slide 18 discusses some of the practicalities of feeding. Units may have differing ideas about when to aspirate nasogastric tubes and the volumes that may suggest difficulties. It is worth making the point that policy in this area will vary between units, and that in some patients, eg those on the ICU, it may be appropriate to try prokinetic agents such as metoclopramide or erythromycin if aspirates are high.

Slide 19 introduces discussion around the need to plan for discontinuation of nasogastric feeding as many surgical trainees do not have experience of planning this.

Scenario 2 (slides 20–32)

This case concerns a woman who developed complications following elective surgery. The discussion centres on total parenteral nutrition (TPN), but **slide 21** makes the point that the choice of method of nutrition should be made at the time of surgery so that appropriate access routes can be obtained.

Slide 22 illustrates some of the important considerations for giving TPN that are illustrated in **slides 24** and **25** (importance of infection control measures, asepsis in preparation and clean administration using a no touch technique).

Slides 26–31 introduce the importance of glycaemic control in all surgical patients. TPN, in particular, can have the effect of raising blood sugar levels in critically ill surgical patients, even those who are non-diabetic.

Slide 29 discusses the original trial illustrating better outcomes from strict glycaemic control (Van den Berge study, **slide 30**) and the difficulties other groups have had in maintaining such tight glycaemic control and the potential harm to patients. NICE-SUGAR (**slide 31**) is now the most widely accepted trial and has been influential in ensuring that blood glucose is maintained in a recommended range of 8–10 mmol/L.

Scenario 3 (slides 32–37)

This case has been chosen to allow discussion of the role of percutaneous endoscopic gastrostomy (PEG)/percutaneous endoscopic jejunostomy (PEJ) feeding and the information that surgical trainees need to know in order to care for patients being fed by PEG. The case is a patient who had complications from nasogastric tubes and needs on-going enteral feeding, but should also be used to make the point and lead a brief discussion about the role of providing a

PEG/PEJ access route at the time of surgery in some patients, eg those undergoing oesophageal surgery. Experience of the group of surgical trainees may be mixed, and it can be helpful to allow some members of the group to share their knowledge with the wider group.

1

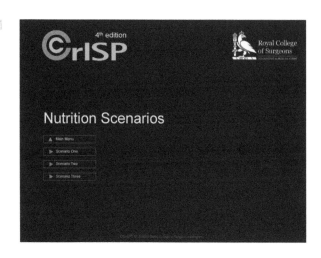

4th edition

CrISP

Royal College of Surgeons

Nutrition Scenarios

- Main Menu
- Scenario One
- Scenario Two
- Scenario Three

2

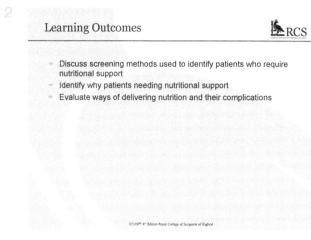

Learning Outcomes RCS

- Discuss screening methods used to identify patients who require nutritional support
- Identify why patients needing nutritional support
- Evaluate ways of delivering nutrition and their complications

3

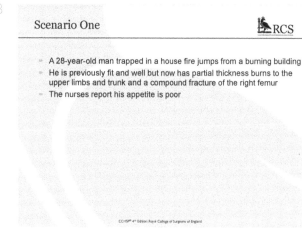

Scenario One RCS

- A 28-year-old man trapped in a house fire jumps from a burning building
- He is previously fit and well but now has partial thickness burns to the upper limbs and trunk and a compound fracture of the right femur
- The nurses report his appetite is poor

4

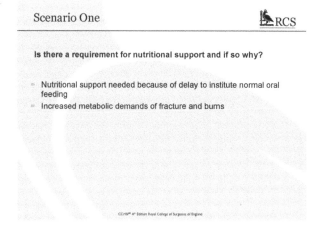

Scenario One RCS

Is there a requirement for nutritional support and if so why?

- Nutritional support needed because of delay to institute normal oral feeding
- Increased metabolic demands of fracture and burns

5

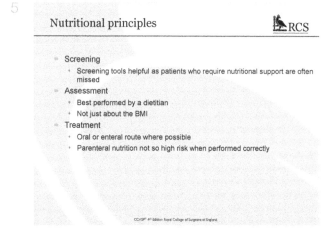

Nutritional principles RCS

- Screening
  - Screening tools helpful as patients who require nutritional support are often missed
- Assessment
  - Best performed by a dietitian
  - Not just about the BMI
- Treatment
  - Oral or enteral route where possible
  - Parenteral nutrition not so high risk when performed correctly

6

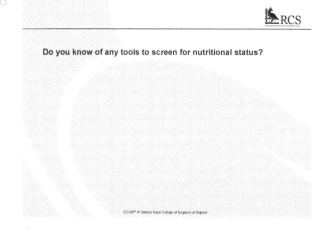

RCS

Do you know of any tools to screen for nutritional status?

7

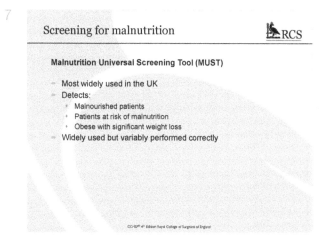

Screening for malnutrition RCS

Malnutrition Universal Screening Tool (MUST)

- Most widely used in the UK
- Detects:
  - Malnourished patients
  - Patients at risk of malnutrition
  - Obese with significant weight loss
- Widely used but variably performed correctly

8

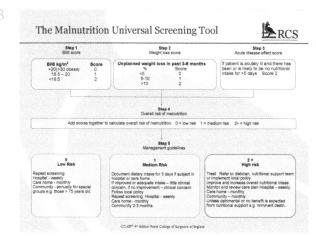

The Malnutrition Universal Screening Tool RCS

9

Nutrition assessment

RCS

- **History**
  - Recent weight loss (5-10% significant)
- **Examination**
  - Anthropometric measures
  - BMI based on weight & height (important to measure)
- **Blood tests**
  - Not particularly helpful. Often a better measure of hydration status and illness
  - Albumin is not a nutritional measure in the sick/hospitalized patient
- **Clinical judgment**
  - Perhaps the most important factor
  - Look at the arms (mid arm)

CCrISP® 4th Edition Royal College of Surgeons of England

10

Weight can be deceptive

RCS

- The weight of ascites and/or oedema needs to be subtracted in order to estimate a dry weight.

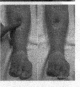

	Ascites (Kg)	Oedema (Kg)
Minimal	2.2	1.0
Moderate	6.0	5.0
Severe	14.0	10.0

CCrISP® 4th Edition Royal College of Surgeons of England

11

Metabolic demands and illness

RCS

What illnesses / conditions increase metabolic demands?

Condition		Stress factor (% BMR)
Infection		25 - 45%
ICU	Ventilated	0 - 10%
	Septic	20 - 60%
Surgery	Uncomplicated	5 - 20%
	Complicated	25 - 40%

CCrISP® 4th Edition Royal College of Surgeons of England

12

Scenario One

RCS

How could you provide nutrition in this man and which route is best?
- Enteral versus parenteral nutrition
- Enteral preferable with intact GI tract
- Oral supplements may be insufficient
- NG route may be preferable

CCrISP® 4th Edition Royal College of Surgeons of England

13

Scenario One

RCS

What are the advantages and disadvantages of NG feeding in this man?

- Advantages
  - Physiological
  - Effective, cheap, safe
  - Less incidence of hyperglycaemia, cholestasis, hypertriglycerideamia
- Disadvantages
  - Difficulty
  - Placing tube or misplacement
  - Obtaining a pH <5.5
  - Pulmonary aspiration
  - Discomfort
  - Pressure necrosis
  - Diarrhoea

CCrISP® 4th Edition Royal College of Surgeons of England

14

NG tube insertion

RCS

- Placed for feeding, administration of medication or gastric decompression

- Misplaced NG tubes can result in respiratory complications and death
  - Listed as a Never Event by the DoH in 2013 as felt to be avoidable (misplacement with feed infused)
  - Consider to be misplaced if the tip is not within the gastro-oesophageal lumen or below the gastro-oesophageal junction
  - Errors in assessment of tube position (pH and CXR)

CCrISP® 4th Edition Royal College of Surgeons of England

15

CALORIES Trial

RCS

- Patients with an unplanned admission to ICU who could be fed enterally or parenterally (33 general ICUs in England).
- Assessed if parenteral is superior to enteral route for the delivery of early nutritional support.
- Primary outcome: all-cause mortality at 30 days.
- Secondary outcomes:
  - Duration of organ support
  - Infectious and non-infectious complications
  - Length of stay (ICU and hospital)
  - Duration of survival
  - Mortality from the ICU and hospital (90 days and 1 year)

Harvey et al. N Engl J Med 2014; 371:1673-1684

CCrISP® 4th Edition Royal College of Surgeons of England

16

CALORIES trial: results

RCS

		Parenteral group	Enteral group	Relative risk	P value
Primary outcome					
Death within 30 days		393/1188 (33.1%)	409/1195 (34.2%)	0.97	0.57
Secondary outcomes					
Duration of organ support					
Infectious comps		0.22 ± 0.6	0.21 ± 0.56		0.72
Non-infectious comps (vomiting)		100/1191 (8.4%)	194/1197 (16.2%)		<0.001
Length of stay	ICU	8.1 (4-15.8)	7.3 (3.9-14.3)		0.15
	Hospital	17 (8-34)	16 (8-33)		0.32
Mortality	ICU	317/1190	352/1197	0.91	0.13
	Hospital	431/1185	4510/1186	0.96	0.44
	90 days	442/1184	464/1188	0.96	0.40

Harvey et al. N Engl J Med 2014; 371:1673-1684

CCrISP® 4th Edition Royal College of Surgeons of England

17

CALORIES trial, take-home messages: 🦁RCS

- No difference in EN or PN in ICU patients
- EN and PN equally effective
- PN not associated with more adverse outcomes

CCrISP® 4ᵗʰ Edition Royal College of Surgeons of England

18

Scenario One 🦁RCS

What are the practicalities of NG feeding in this man?

- Nurse at 30-45 degrees head up
- Use a protocol e.g. 30ml/h, aspirate after 4 hours
- Gastric volumes
- Decide volumes to continue feed (<200-300ml)
- Gastroparesis is common (medications / blood flow / illness)
- If poor gastric emptying then jejunal feeding can be considered (but do not delay nutrition support)
- Consider prokinetics if volumes are excessive

CCrISP® 4ᵗʰ Edition Royal College of Surgeons of England

19

Scenario One 🦁RCS

When would you wean off NG feeding?

- Patient eating and drinking
- Introduce normal diet during the day and continue with nocturnal NG feeding
- Reduce night feeds as daytime feeding increases
- Supplement daytime diet
- Record nutritional intake
- Involve dietician/nutrition team

CCrISP® 4ᵗʰ Edition Royal College of Surgeons of England

20

Scenario Two 🦁RCS

- A 75-year-old woman is admitted for elective reversal of a Hartmann's procedure
- The operation is difficult and complicated by adhesions, so that she has to return to theatre 5 days later due to intra-abdominal sepsis
- She has an anastomotic leak and another Hartmann's is performed
- She is taken to ICU post operatively

CCrISP® 4ᵗʰ Edition Royal College of Surgeons of England

21

Scenario Two 🦁RCS

How should we give this woman nutrition?

- **Gastric**
  - NG unlikely to be tolerated (gastroparesis)
- **Jejunal**
  - NJ unlikely to be tolerated (ileus)
- **Parenteral nutrition**
  - PN best option: she is unlikely to resume normal nutrition for some time
  - Dedicated clean CV access
  - .Single / multilumen CVC or PICC

CCrISP® 4ᵗʰ Edition Royal College of Surgeons of England

22

Scenario Two 🦁RCS

What are the practicalities of giving TPN?

- Dedicated CVC
  - 1 lumen of multilumen CVC
  - Single lumen CVC
  - PICC
  - Tunneled cuffed CVC
- Strict asepsis catheter care (medications and nutrition)
- Fluid balance chart
- 'Routine' observations
- Daily weights
- Daily inspection of CVC exit site
- Monitor glycaemic control: daily urinalysis, other chemistry
- Do not restart same feed once bag has been disconnected

CCrISP® 4ᵗʰ Edition Royal College of Surgeons of England

23

Parenteral nutrition 🦁RCS

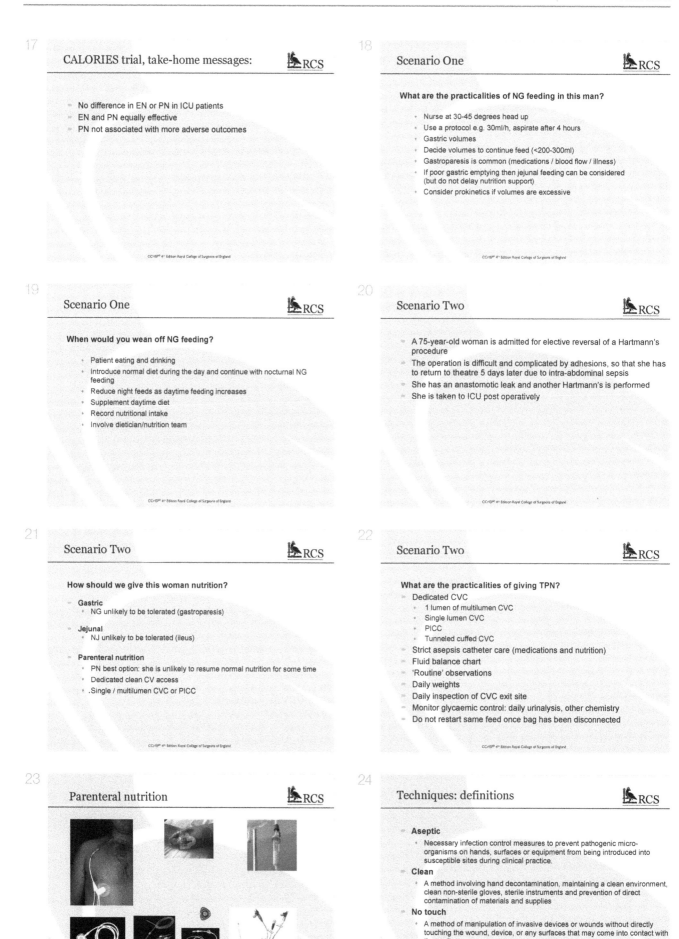

CCrISP® 4ᵗʰ Edition Royal College of Surgeons of England

24

Techniques: definitions 🦁RCS

- **Aseptic**
  - Necessary infection control measures to prevent pathogenic micro-organisms on hands, surfaces or equipment from being introduced into susceptible sites during clinical practice.
- **Clean**
  - A method involving hand decontamination, maintaining a clean environment, clean non-sterile gloves, sterile instruments and prevention of direct contamination of materials and supplies
- **No touch**
  - A method of manipulation of invasive devices or wounds without directly touching the wound, device, or any surfaces that may come into contact with those sites.

Dougherty et al (2010)   Association for Professionals in Infection Control and Epidemiology (2001)

CCrISP® 4ᵗʰ Edition Royal College of Surgeons of England

25

Aseptic Non Touch Technique

RCS

- Peer reviewed and tested clinical guidelines
  - Basic infection prevention and control principles
- Aim to standardise and improve the efficacy of the aseptic technique thereby reducing healthcare associated infections
  - Standard or surgical depending on length and complexity of procedure (Rowley, 1994 and 2004)

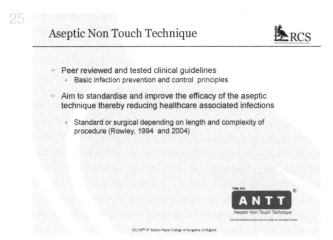

26

The metabolic role of insulin

RCS

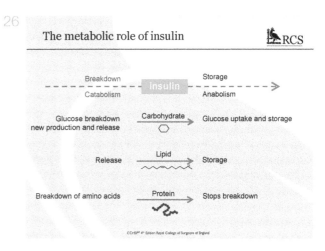

27

Insulin Resistance

RCS

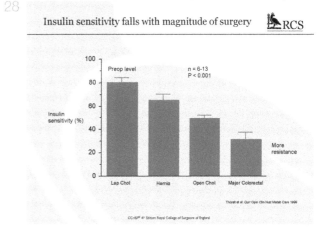

28

Insulin sensitivity falls with magnitude of surgery

RCS

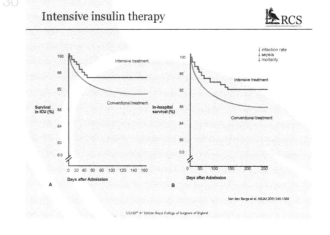

29

Glycaemic control in critical illness

RCS

- Hyperglycemia is common in critical illness
  - 90% develop blood glucose > 6.1 mmol/L
- Landmark trials:
  - Van den Berge (NEJM 2001): targeted normoglycemia (4.4-6.1 mmol/L) reduced mortality and morbidity
  - NICE-SUGAR (NEJM 2009): increased mortality with this approach
  - SPRINT (Crit Care, 2008): computerised glucose modeling reduced mortality
- Recommendations now are for a more moderate blood glucose target of 8-10 mmol/L

30

Intensive insulin therapy

RCS

31

NICE-SUGAR Study Intensive v conventional glucose control

RCS

32

Scenario Three

RCS

- A 32-year-old man was involved in a road traffic collision during which he sustained a severe head injury
- He was discharged from ICU with a tracheostomy and is nasogastrically fed (he did not have a basal skull fracture)
- He still has impaired swallowing and a poor gag reflex but the nasogastric tube is causing ulceration of his nasal septum

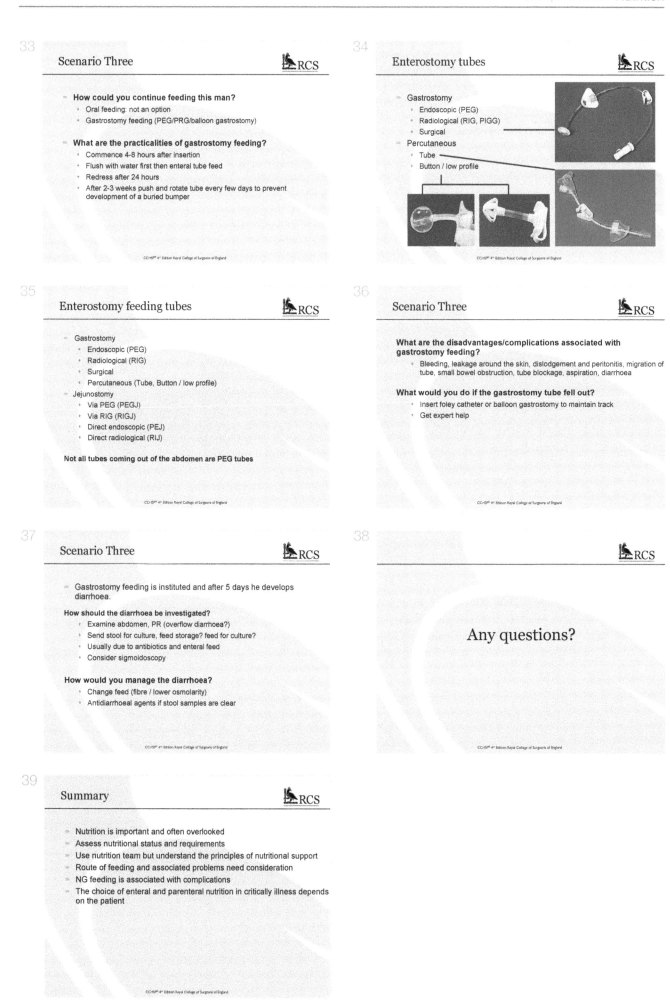

33

Scenario Three

- How could you continue feeding this man?
  - Oral feeding: not an option
  - Gastrostomy feeding (PEG/PRG/balloon gastrostomy)

- What are the practicalities of gastrostomy feeding?
  - Commence 4-8 hours after insertion
  - Flush with water first then enteral tube feed
  - Redress after 24 hours
  - After 2-3 weeks push and rotate tube every few days to prevent development of a buried bumper

34

Enterostomy tubes

- Gastrostomy
  - Endoscopic (PEG)
  - Radiological (RIG, PIGG)
  - Surgical
- Percutaneous
  - Tube
  - Button / low profile

35

Enterostomy feeding tubes

- Gastrostomy
  - Endoscopic (PEG)
  - Radiological (RIG)
  - Surgical
  - Percutaneous (Tube, Button / low profile)
- Jejunostomy
  - Via PEG (PEGJ)
  - Via RIG (RIGJ)
  - Direct endoscopic (PEJ)
  - Direct radiological (RIJ)

Not all tubes coming out of the abdomen are PEG tubes

36

Scenario Three

What are the disadvantages/complications associated with gastrostomy feeding?
  - Bleeding, leakage around the skin, dislodgement and peritonitis, migration of tube, small bowel obstruction, tube blockage, aspiration, diarrhoea

What would you do if the gastrostomy tube fell out?
  - Insert foley catheter or balloon gastrostomy to maintain track
  - Get expert help

37

Scenario Three

- Gastrostomy feeding is instituted and after 5 days he develops diarrhoea.

How should the diarrhoea be investigated?
  - Examine abdomen, PR (overflow diarrhoea?)
  - Send stool for culture, feed storage? feed for culture?
  - Usually due to antibiotics and enteral feed
  - Consider sigmoidoscopy

How would you manage the diarrhoea?
  - Change feed (fibre / lower osmolarity)
  - Antidiarrhoeal agents if stool samples are clear

38

Any questions?

39

Summary

- Nutrition is important and often overlooked
- Assess nutritional status and requirements
- Use nutrition team but understand the principles of nutritional support
- Route of feeding and associated problems need consideration
- NG feeding is associated with complications
- The choice of enteral and parenteral nutrition in critically illness depends on the patient

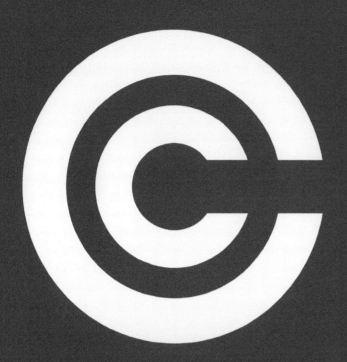

2.0

Small group session
The unwell surgical patient

Overview

In this session the candidates are taken through three cases of patients with sepsis. The aim is to illustrate how the three-stage assessment system can be used to recognise deteriorating patients and to work out the reason for the deterioration. The material has been presented in a way that tries to stick to the CCrISP assessment system as far as is possible with a workshop exercise.

The cases are based on actual patients and are presented in slightly different ways in an attempt to make the candidates think a bit harder while still encouraging use of the CCrISP assessment system. The idea is to try to get the candidates to imagine what they would be thinking and feeling if these were real-life situations. It is important that all the data interpretation is done by the candidates with minimal prompting from the instructor, otherwise the opportunity to explore the candidates' understanding and to get them to help each other is lost. Questions and tasks for the candidates appear on the slides to help faculty follow the logic of the cases and to aid running the session.

It may not be possible to get through all three cases: case 1 is designed to take the most time and case 3 the least as the principles of sepsis management should have been established in case 1 discussion.

Duration	45 minutes
Style	Small group interactive discussion
AV	PowerPoint presentation

Learning outcomes

By the end of the session, participants should be able to:

- evaluate the utility of the three-stage assessment process in managing unwell patients;

- formulate plans to treat abnormal patient physiology;

- formulate a unifying explanation for a patient's deterioration;

- understand their role in the management of patients at risk of poor outcomes.

Scenario 1

This is a case of an elective recurrent incisional hernia repair in a patient with significant comorbidities. There is essentially a failure to progress, which, it could be argued, is recognised a bit late.

Slides 3–7 set the scene and go through the immediate management and full patient assessment. There is lot of information here, as would be the case with a real-life patient, and the aim is to get the candidates to draw out the important details and to weight them accordingly. It could be argued that the choice of operation is unusual, and it may be worth discussing this at the appropriate point (**slide 17**, do not waste time discussing the nuances of surgical technique at the expense of emphasising the treatment of sepsis). It should be noted that the patient is still in hospital 6 days after the surgery, is still on a morphine PCA and is failing to progress and that an explanation for these observations needs to be found.

Slides 9–11 go through the new sepsis definitions (February 2016). The new definitions move away from the importance of recognising systemic inflammatory response syndrome to trying to recognise as early as possible the group of patients in whom outcomes are poorer. Many patients with systemic inflammatory response syndrome and an infection do not have poor outcomes; this does not mean that this group of patients is unimportant, but significant improvements in outcomes will not come from focusing on this group. Sepsis is defined as the suspicion of infection in the presence of organ dysfunction (severe sepsis in the previous nomenclature). The recommendation is that organ dysfunction is detected using the sequential organ failure assessment (SOFA) methodology, but as this is really suited only to an ITU setting, and the aim is to detect sepsis at an earlier stage, a modification of this, quick SOFA (qSOFA), has been advocated. qSOFA encompasses respiratory rate >22, systolic BP <100 mmHg and altered mental state; the presence of each scores 1 point, and sepsis should be suspected if the score is 2 or more. This score can also equate to abnormal scoring on the NEWS and, although formal guidance has not yet been published at the time of writing, it is expected that NICE will recommend using NEWS instead of qSOFA.

Severe sepsis is defined as failure to respond rapidly to fluid resuscitation and, once this is recognised, intensive care support should be enlisted promptly, if not already done. The mechanism for doing this will differ from hospital to hospital depending on the local set-up, and it may be useful to discuss this with the candidates to ensure that they understand how their hospital functions and what their role is.

Slides 12–17 return to the scenario and go through more data and interpretation, culminating in a chance to reflect on the whole case with the group; for example, **slide 13** (ABG result) shows a subtle abnormality of blood lactate level while **slide 14** shows a raised white cell count (WCC) and international normalised ratio (INR), reduced platelet count, and evidence of development of acute kidney injury (AKI). The patient did not respond to initial treatment, was transferred back to the HDU and returned to theatre for a laparotomy. A small bowel perforation was found, damage limitation surgery was carried out and a laparostoma created. The patient survived after a prolonged ITU and hospital stay.

Slide 17 is optional – feel free to omit it.

Scenario 2

This case is introduced in a slightly different way by giving more of the information about the patient first; the case should still be discussed with the three-stage assessment process in mind, resisting the temptation to allow the candidates to jump to conclusions.

Slides 18 and **19** describe a patient who is admitted with adhesive small bowel obstruction, confirmed on CT, and who is initially treated conservatively.

Slide 20 sets the scene for the candidates to become involved; the patient starts scoring on the track and trigger system.

Slides 21–23 provide data that the candidates should interpret, and they should realise that more information is needed. Various suggestions may be made at this stage, but the main piece of missing information is previous blood results for comparison. This is intended to put the candidates into the scenario and to think through the process, as in real clinical practice they would have to request and chase up investigations. The additional subtlety in these results is the low WCC, which, when allied to the raised INR, lactate and possible AKI, should flag up deterioration and the question of sepsis, even without previous results for comparison.

Slides 24 and **25** ask a series of questions and then take the candidates through the rationale of the thinking and decision-making.

Slide 25 concludes the scenario by outlining what happened in this case. There was no other obvious source of sepsis, but there was definite abdominal pathology that was failing to respond to conservative treatment, so laparotomy was justified. The merits of preoperative CT could be discussed if there is time.

Scenario 3

Scenario 3 starts (**slide 27**) by setting the scene for the candidates' involvement with the case. Do not labour the use of the three-stage assessment process if the candidates have already demonstrated they are following the principles.

Slide 28 gives more information. The patient needs continued high-flow oxygen therapy and fluid resuscitation with fluid challenges and reassessment. Candidates should immediately realise that this patient differs from the previous two as she has presented with more advanced pathology and should recognise that speed and accuracy of treatment are of vital importance.

Slides 29–31 provide more data for interpretation and discussion together with some questions aimed at obtaining all the information that is needed. Important points from **slide 30** are the raised WBC, the significant renal dysfunction and the missing K^+ result, which will need to be obtained urgently as the patient may well be hyperkalaemic (put in to emphasise attention to detail).

Slide 32 shows a marked acidosis, relative hypoxia and a markedly raised lactate, indicating the severe nature of this patient's condition. This should be picked up by the candidates and should add to the urgency with which the patient should be treated and the speed with which her level of care should be escalated.

Slide 33 brings together where the candidates have reached in their management plan. There are multiple possibilities for the source of the sepsis, and each should be considered in turn, including the need for cerebrospinal fluid (CSF) sampling as an infected ventriculoperitoneal shunt is a possibility. The blisters on the skin should prompt the consideration of necrotising fasciitis. This patient had a bladder stone and this was a presentation, along with urosepsis. These details can be revealed at the end of the case but are not necessary to bring out the learning objectives.

Slide 34 presents questions and **slide 35** summarises of the learning objectives of the session.

Timeline

Introduction	2 minutes
Scenario 1	15 minutes
Scenario 2	13 minutes
Scenario 3	10 minutes
Questions and summary	5 minutes

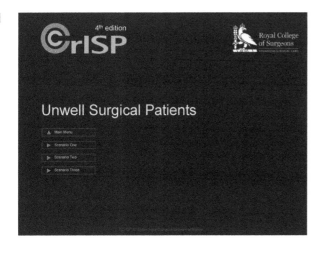

Learning Outcomes

- Evaluate the utility of the 3 stage assessment process in managing unwell patients
- Formulate plans to support abnormal physiology
- Formulate a unifying explanation for a patient's deterioration
- Understand your role in the management of patients at risk of poor outcomes

Scenario One

At the morning handover the night FY2 tells you of a 63 year old man who she saw overnight because he was unwell. He underwent a recurrent incisional hernia repair 6 days ago, went to HDU post op and is now back on the ward. You prioritise this patient for review immediately after handover.

How will you approach this problem?

Initial Assessment

A Patent
B RR 22, poor inspiratory effort, bilateral basal crepitations, O_2 sats 94% on room air
C CRT 4 secs, P 110 reg, BP 90/60
D Confused, pupils normal, BM 5.8 mmol/l
E PCA in situ, good IV access left forearm, abdomen distended, temp 38.3°C

What parameters are of concern?
How will you treat this initially?
What will you do next?

Full Patient Assessment

Notes review (key points)
- 63 year old male, 177 cm, 106 kg BMI 33.8
- Hartmann's procedure for perforated diverticular disease 6 years ago
- Incisional hernia repair 4 years ago
- Abdominal pain since initial op, recurrent hernia diagnosed 2 years ago
- Hypertension, COPD, Obstructive Sleep Apnoea,
- former smoker, 10 units alcohol/week
- Seen in clinic 4 months ago (SpR, listed for elective incisional hernia repair)
- 6 days ago Incisional Hernia Repair – see op note

Full Patient Assessment – Op note

Operation Description
- Laparoscopy and division of adhesions, recurrent incisional hernia repair with component separation and mesh insertion.

Procedure
- Multiple defects in the midline
- Pneumoperitoneum created and laparoscope inserted without incident
- Extensive adhesiolysis to reduce the contents of hernial sac
- 1 small serosal tear made in the small bowel – closed with 3.0 vicryl
- No contamination
- Midline laparotomy without entering the abdominal cavity. Rectus sheath releasing incision to release tension. Pre-peritoneal space created for mesh – 5cm overlap
- Hernial defects closed in midline with 3 O nylon
- Preperitoneal mesh 30 x 20cm x 1 sutured to fascia with 2-O Ethibond
- Redivac drain 16 F x 3-10 Fr x 1 to wound (in front of mesh)
- Good haemostasis

Post-op
- Patient to HDU, fluids and diet as tolerated, drain to stay until further notice

Full Patient Assessment – Post op progress

Day 1 Obs stable, PCA, paracetamol and ibuprofen, CPAP
Day 2 Obs stable, patient complaining of pain, not mobilising
Day 3 Vomiting bile stained fluid, 650 ml fluid from drains, abdomen distended, no flatus or bowel action, IVI to continue, ng tube inserted.
Day 4 No further vomiting, ng losses 500 mls.
Day 5 SaO_2 93% on 3L/min O_2, HR 83, T 36°C, RR 18, BP 127/80

WC 9.7, U 8.8. Plan ng spigotted, erythromycin and metoclopramide started, consider TPN

What is of concern here?
What is the next step?

Decide and Plan

Patient not making expected progress.

What is the explanation?

Could this be sepsis?

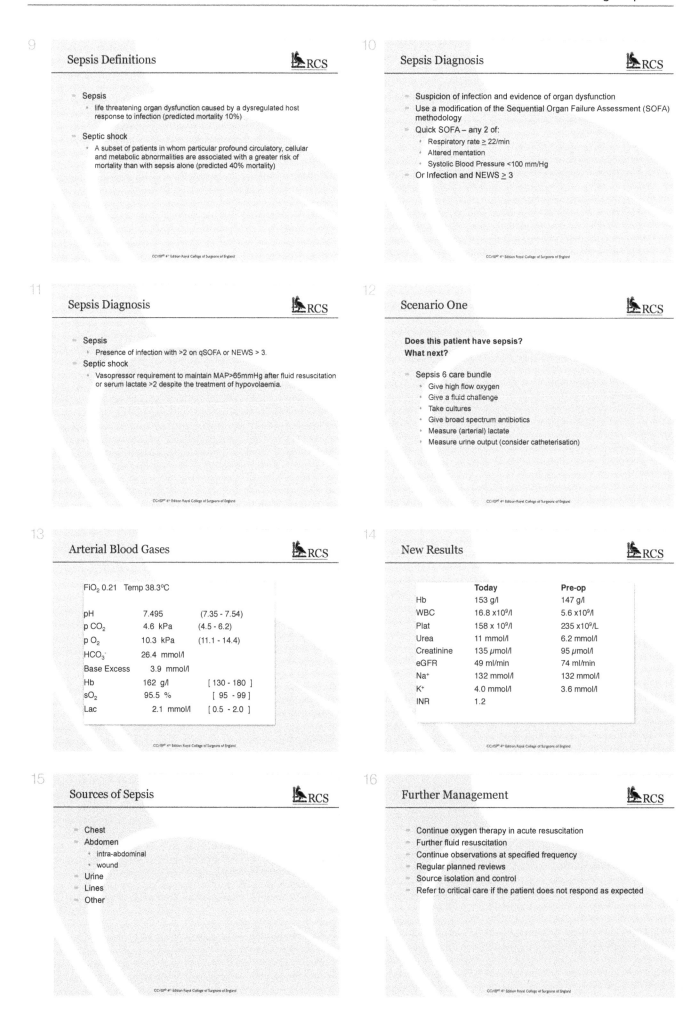

9

Sepsis Definitions RCS

- Sepsis
  - life threatening organ dysfunction caused by a dysregulated host response to infection (predicted mortality 10%)

- Septic shock
  - A subset of patients in whom particular profound circulatory, cellular and metabolic abnormalities are associated with a greater risk of mortality than with sepsis alone (predicted 40% mortality)

CCrISP® 4th Edition Royal College of Surgeons of England

10

Sepsis Diagnosis RCS

- Suspicion of infection and evidence of organ dysfunction
- Use a modification of the Sequential Organ Failure Assessment (SOFA) methodology
- Quick SOFA – any 2 of:
  - Respiratory rate ≥ 22/min
  - Altered mentation
  - Systolic Blood Pressure <100 mm/Hg
- Or Infection and NEWS ≥ 3

CCrISP® 4th Edition Royal College of Surgeons of England

11

Sepsis Diagnosis RCS

- Sepsis
  - Presence of infection with >2 on qSOFA or NEWS > 3.
- Septic shock
  - Vasopressor requirement to maintain MAP>65mmHg after fluid resuscitation or serum lactate >2 despite the treatment of hypovolaemia.

CCrISP® 4th Edition Royal College of Surgeons of England

12

Scenario One RCS

Does this patient have sepsis?
What next?

- Sepsis 6 care bundle
  - Give high flow oxygen
  - Give a fluid challenge
  - Take cultures
  - Give broad spectrum antibiotics
  - Measure (arterial) lactate
  - Measure urine output (consider catheterisation)

CCrISP® 4th Edition Royal College of Surgeons of England

13

Arterial Blood Gases RCS

FiO$_2$ 0.21   Temp 38.3°C

pH	7.495	(7.35 - 7.54)
p CO$_2$	4.6 kPa	(4.5 - 6.2)
p O$_2$	10.3 kPa	(11.1 - 14.4)
HCO$_3^-$	26.4 mmol/l	
Base Excess	3.9 mmol/l	
Hb	162 g/l	[130 - 180]
sO$_2$	95.5 %	[95 - 99]
Lac	2.1 mmol/l	[0.5 - 2.0]

CCrISP® 4th Edition Royal College of Surgeons of England

14

New Results RCS

	Today	Pre-op
Hb	153 g/l	147 g/l
WBC	16.8 x10^9/l	5.6 x10^9/l
Plat	158 x 10^9/l	235 x10^9/L
Urea	11 mmol/l	6.2 mmol/l
Creatinine	135 μmol/l	95 μmol/l
eGFR	49 ml/min	74 ml/min
Na$^+$	132 mmol/l	132 mmol/l
K$^+$	4.0 mmol/l	3.6 mmol/l
INR	1.2	

CCrISP® 4th Edition Royal College of Surgeons of England

15

Sources of Sepsis RCS

- Chest
- Abdomen
  - intra-abdominal
  - wound
- Urine
- Lines
- Other

CCrISP® 4th Edition Royal College of Surgeons of England

16

Further Management RCS

- Continue oxygen therapy in acute resuscitation
- Further fluid resuscitation
- Continue observations at specified frequency
- Regular planned reviews
- Source isolation and control
- Refer to critical care if the patient does not respond as expected

CCrISP® 4th Edition Royal College of Surgeons of England

17

Whole Case Review 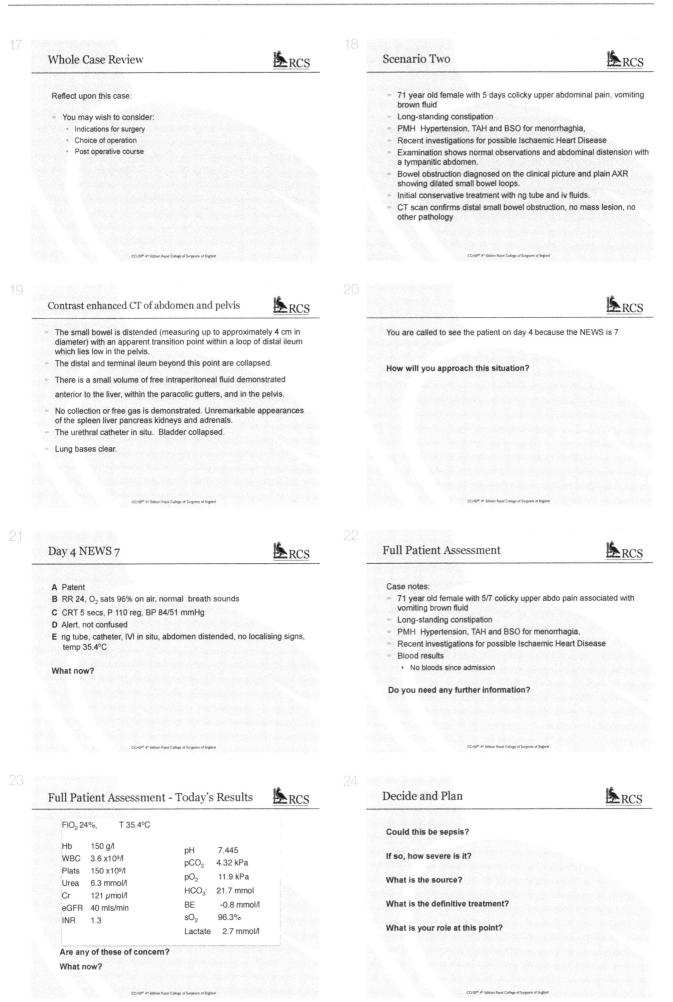 RCS

Reflect upon this case:

- You may wish to consider:
  - Indications for surgery
  - Choice of operation
  - Post operative course

CCrISP® 4ᵗʰ Edition Royal College of Surgeons of England

18

Scenario Two RCS

- 71 year old female with 5 days colicky upper abdominal pain, vomiting brown fluid
- Long-standing constipation
- PMH Hypertension, TAH and BSO for menorrhaghia,
- Recent investigations for possible Ischaemic Heart Disease
- Examination shows normal observations and abdominal distension with a tympanitic abdomen.
- Bowel obstruction diagnosed on the clinical picture and plain AXR showing dilated small bowel loops.
- Initial conservative treatment with ng tube and iv fluids.
- CT scan confirms distal small bowel obstruction, no mass lesion, no other pathology

CCrISP® 4ᵗʰ Edition Royal College of Surgeons of England

19

Contrast enhanced CT of abdomen and pelvis RCS

- The small bowel is distended (measuring up to approximately 4 cm in diameter) with an apparent transition point within a loop of distal ileum which lies low in the pelvis.
- The distal and terminal ileum beyond this point are collapsed.
- There is a small volume of free intraperitoneal fluid demonstrated anterior to the liver, within the paracolic gutters, and in the pelvis.
- No collection or free gas is demonstrated. Unremarkable appearances of the spleen liver pancreas kidneys and adrenals.
- The urethral catheter in situ. Bladder collapsed.
- Lung bases clear.

CCrISP® 4ᵗʰ Edition Royal College of Surgeons of England

20

RCS

You are called to see the patient on day 4 because the NEWS is 7

How will you approach this situation?

CCrISP® 4ᵗʰ Edition Royal College of Surgeons of England

21

Day 4 NEWS 7 RCS

A Patent
B RR 24, O₂ sats 96% on air, normal breath sounds
C CRT 5 secs, P 110 reg, BP 84/51 mmHg
D Alert, not confused
E ng tube, catheter, IVI in situ, abdomen distended, no localising signs, temp 35.4°C

What now?

CCrISP® 4ᵗʰ Edition Royal College of Surgeons of England

22

Full Patient Assessment RCS

Case notes:
- 71 year old female with 5/7 colicky upper abdo pain associated with vomiting brown fluid
- Long-standing constipation
- PMH Hypertension, TAH and BSO for menorrhagia,
- Recent investigations for possible Ischaemic Heart Disease
- Blood results
  - No bloods since admission

Do you need any further information?

CCrISP® 4ᵗʰ Edition Royal College of Surgeons of England

23

Full Patient Assessment - Today's Results RCS

FiO₂ 24%,   T 35.4°C

Hb	150 g/l	pH	7.445
WBC	3.6 x10⁹/l	pCO₂	4.32 kPa
Plats	150 x10⁹/l	pO₂	11.9 kPa
Urea	6.3 mmol/l	HCO₃⁻	21.7 mmol
Cr	121 μmol/l	BE	-0.8 mmol/l
eGFR	40 mls/min	sO₂	96.3%
INR	1.3	Lactate	2.7 mmol/l

Are any of these of concern?
What now?

CCrISP® 4ᵗʰ Edition Royal College of Surgeons of England

24

Decide and Plan RCS

Could this be sepsis?

If so, how severe is it?

What is the source?

What is the definitive treatment?

What is your role at this point?

CCrISP® 4ᵗʰ Edition Royal College of Surgeons of England

25

Rationale   RCS

- Infection suspected (WBC, low temp)
- qSOFA 2, NEWS >3
- 'Sepsis 6' bundle needs completing
- Insufficient information to decide if this is severe sepsis at this stage.
- Possibility of new organ dysfunction
- Consider the "surgical sources". Definite intra-abdominal pathology in this case but appears to be uncomplicated SBO given the radiology
- This previously stable patient has deteriorated. Your role is to recognise this, understand the decisions that need to be made and who should make them.

CCrISP® 4ᵗʰ Edition Royal College of Surgeons of England

26

Subsequent Progress   RCS

Laparotomy

- SBO secondary to a tight band adhesion, perforation at the site of the band with distal small bowel content throughout the lower abdomen

- Resected with primary anastomosis

CCrISP® 4ᵗʰ Edition Royal College of Surgeons of England

27

Scenario Three   RCS

You are called to the Emergency Department to see a patient who the ED staff are concerned about. They say she is very unwell and she has multiple sclerosis.

CCrISP® 4ᵗʰ Edition Royal College of Surgeons of England

28

Immediate Management   RCS

A Patent
B RR 26 on high flow O_2, unrecordable SaO_2
C CRT > 6s, peripherally cyanosed, P122 reg, BP 84/50, some generalised oedema
D responds to voice, confused, obviously unwell
E Abdomen soft, suprapubic catheter, old surgical scar with blisters around it, temperature 37.5°C

What immediate treatment is needed?

CCrISP® 4ᵗʰ Edition Royal College of Surgeons of England

29

Full Patient Assessment   RCS

- 68 year old female presenting feeling hot with a rash. Husband states similar to episode of meningococcal sepsis she had previously.
- He says high temperature, skin rash, weak for 2 days. Complaining of headache.
- PMH Ventriculo-peritoneal shunt 9 years ago for obstructive hydrocephalus
- Multiple Sclerosis with an indwelling suprapubic catheter
- Grade 2 sacral pressure sore
- No current medications
- Allergic to penicillin and trimethoprim
- Lives at home, uses wheelchair and Zimmer Frame, washes and dresses with assistance

CCrISP® 4ᵗʰ Edition Royal College of Surgeons of England

30

Full Patient Assessment - Results   RCS

Hb	113 g/l
WBC	29 x10⁹/l
Plats	187 x10⁹/l
Urea	18.3 mmol/l
Cr	480 μmol/l
eGFR	8 ml/min
Na⁺	143
K⁺	Haemolysed
Bil	9 mmol/l
ALT	65 iu/l
Alk P	288 iu/l

What are the relevant abnormal results?
What's next?

CCrISP® 4ᵗʰ Edition Royal College of Surgeons of England

31

Decide and Plan   RCS

- This lady meets the criteria for sepsis
  - suspected infection, altered mental state, raised respiratory rate, hypotension.

What other blood test is needed?
  - ABG

What are the potential sources of sepsis in this patient?
  - Chest
  - Abdomen
  - Urinary tract
  - Neuro
  - Skin

How will you proceed now?

CCrISP® 4ᵗʰ Edition Royal College of Surgeons of England

32

Further Results   RCS

- CXR poor inspiratory effort, no focal consolidation
- CT head: consistent with previous treatment, no new pathology
- ABG (on high flow oxygen)
  - pH   7.25
  - pCO_2 3.5 kPa
  - pO_2 10.1 kPa
  - HCO_3^- 11.1 mmol/l
  - BE   -14.4 mmol/l
  - Lactate   11.7 mmol/l

How do you interpret these results?
What do you need to do now?

CCrISP® 4ᵗʰ Edition Royal College of Surgeons of England

33

Summary of Management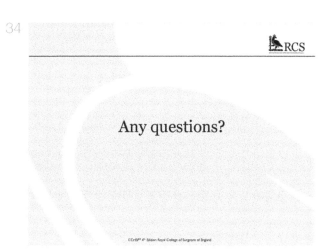

- Continue to administer high flow O_2
- Serial fluid challenges
- Take appropriate cultures including blood cultures
- Administer antibiotics. What would you cover?
- Start measuring urine output
- Escalate to critical care now

CCrISP® 4th Edition Royal College of Surgeons of England

34

Any questions?

CCrISP® 4th Edition Royal College of Surgeons of England

35

Summary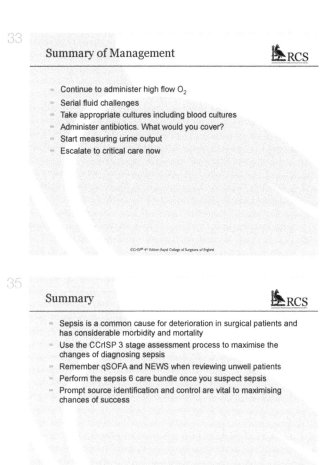

- Sepsis is a common cause for deterioration in surgical patients and has considerable morbidity and mortality
- Use the CCrISP 3 stage assessment process to maximise the changes of diagnosing sepsis
- Remember qSOFA and NEWS when reviewing unwell patients
- Perform the sepsis 6 care bundle once you suspect sepsis
- Prompt source identification and control are vital to maximising chances of success

CCrISP® 4th Edition Royal College of Surgeons of England

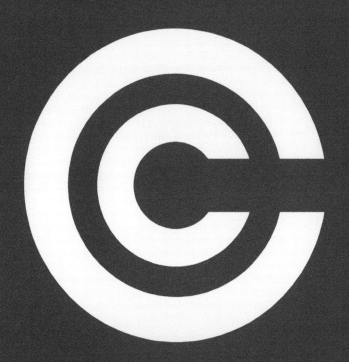

Small group session
Ward dilemmas

Introduction

This session explores some of the difficulties associated with surgical decision-making, particularly in patients who may be approaching the end of their life.

The intention is to set the scene by outlining the session's learning objectives and then to lead an interactive discussion, taking the participants through two scenarios that encompass consideration of futility, end-of-life care, consent, DNACPR (do not attempt cardiopulmonary resuscitation) and associated communications.

The theme that runs through the session is one of lack of absolute certainty and 'shades of grey' in surgical care. The following should be emphasised:

   Appropriate patient care does not necessarily include a full panoply of active treatments.

   CPR is a form of treatment that may not be appropriate at the end of life. Resuscitation includes the basics of oxygen, intravenous fluids and antibiotics. **Decisions concerning withdrawal of 'life-prolonging' treatments do not equate to 'do not care'** and it is best practice to involve the patient, family and other care-givers in these discussions.

   To many people 'a good death', ie one without pain, unnecessary suffering, etc, is very important.

If participants have an understanding of ethical and medico-legal considerations within their country, instructors can use their experiences as a means of leading the discussion, although care should be taken to manage time appropriately.

Duration	45 minutes
Style	Small group interactive discussion
Faculty	Two (as a preference; ideally one surgeon and one anaesthetist/intensivist)
AV	PowerPoint presentation

Learning outcomes

At the end of this session, participants will be able to:

   evaluate the need for holistic elements in surgical care, ie review when surgery is not always the best option;

   formulate the components of care for the dying patient;

   adopt an ethical framework for decision-making in surgical care;

   characterise the uncertainties in patient care.

Scenario 1 (slides 3–23)

Slides 3–6

This scenario deals with a seriously ill female patient with small bowel obstruction and a background of recurrent gynaecological malignancy. The initial part of the scenario utilises the three-stage assessment process.

Slide 7–14

Full patient assessment reveals a supraventricular tachycardia, most probably due to electrolyte imbalances. X-rays demonstrate probable pleural effusions and dilated loops of bowel. CT findings are grossly abnormal (full report below) and haematology and biochemistry parameters are deranged and indicative of probable AKI, liver failure and associated severe metabolic acidaemia.

CT report (portal venous phase scan of the abdomen and pelvis)

- Left hydronephrosis with hydroureter with distal ureteric obstruction.

- 10 cm irregular mass posterior and inseparable from the bladder, rectum and several loops of small bowel consistent with tumour.

- Bilateral iliac nodal metastases and a small amount of ascites.

- 3 cm partially cystic mass in the spleen suspicious of a metastasis.

- Bilateral pleural effusions presumably due to pleural involvement.

Conclusion

- Ovarian carcinoma with widespread pelvic disease involving the bladder, rectum and small bowel. Nodal and probable splenic and pleural metastases. Left hydronephrosis secondary to pelvic ureter involvement by tumour.

Slides 15–17

The final part of the three-stage assessment considers whether or not active treatments are appropriate. The possibility of death should be raised with candidates if they do not mention this themselves.

Slides 18 and 19

Candidates should be encouraged to consider what information doctors need to allow them to act in patients' best interests and discuss whether or not a patient is dying and what their wishes may be. This is an important part of the full patient assessment and is vital for appropriate decision-making and planning.

Consider the definitions of futility from a scientific and holistic perspective before discussing the four fundamentals of medical ethics: **beneficence, non-maleficence, autonomy and distributive justice**.

Many clinicians are guided by these four fundamental principles; debate therefore considers potential conflict between them and how they can be applied case by case. The desire to perform altruistic acts frequently drives healthcare professionals to save lives but, if a patient has been recognised as dying, interventions such as surgery may be futile and subject individuals to 'inhuman and degrading' treatments that can become harmful or maleficent. Thus, despite a desire to honour autonomous wishes and a patient's desire to live, prolonging treatments may infringe the rights of a dying patient by preventing a good death.

At this point candidates can be encouraged to consider life as a philosophical as well as a physiological entity, ie keeping a patient alive may prevent a good death: many cultural and religious contexts view death as a step towards the afterlife or reincarnation. Thus, enabling a 'good death' may not only avoid futile, degrading treatments but also provide the circumstances for the final part of a fulfilling life and protect the religious rights and freedoms of the dying patient as well as the rights and freedoms of other patients requiring treatment (distributive justice). In countries that have signed the European Convention on Human Rights instructors may wish to consider the discussion in the context of Articles 2, 3 and 8 (see below).

In order to minimise delays and prevent discussions being prolonged because of uncertainty or candidates' deeply held personal beliefs, instructors are encouraged to emphasise that patients are considered on a case-by-case basis and (when there is controversy) formal channels for debate exist, including second/third opinions, clinical ethics committees, hospital religious advisors/chaplains and (rarely) *recourse to legal action* in countries' supreme/high courts.

Slides 22 and **23** deal with the provision of end-of-life care. The principles and provisions listed are universal and regarded as being acceptable across most cultures, societies and religions.

This sets the scene and outlines a provisional plan to take a patient who apparently lacks capacity to the operating room for expedited surgery for a limb- and possibly life-threatening condition.

The concept of capacity can be debated (drawing on the Mental Capacity Act 2005 in England and Wales or other relevant legislation for your area), emphasising that mental health problems do not necessarily affect the patient's capacity to consent to surgery and that varying levels of capacity exist.

Slides 26 and 27

The reasons for the improvement in capacity in this patient are uncertain but it could be due to effective analgesia, or control of pyrexia. The fact that several medical experts (including a psychiatrist) have assessed the patient and deemed her to have capacity should be used as the point to move on to the discussion surrounding informed refusal and what the duties of a doctor are in such circumstances.

Slide 28

The scenario encourages discussion about how to manage the patient in accordance with her final decision, eg standard care if she choses surgery or referral to the pain team for palliative care if she continues to refuse surgery. An appropriate advanced care plan can then be developed by the palliative care team in a process of shared decision-making.

Timeline

Introduction and objectives	5 minutes
Scenario 1	25 minutes
Scenario 2	10–12 minutes
Questions and summary	3 minutes

References to assist instructors with preparation

Association of Anaesthetists of Great Britain and Ireland. *Do Not Attempt Resuscitation (DNAR) Decisions in the Perioperative Period*. London: AAGBI; 2009.

Beauchamp T, Childress J. *Principles of Biomedical Ethics*, 4th edn. Oxford: Oxford University Press; 1994.

Callahan D. Living and dying with medical technology. *Crit Care Med* 2003; **31** (5 Suppl.): S344–346.

Cosgrove JF, Nesbitt ID, Bartley C. Futility and the critically ill adult patient. *Curr. Anaes Crit Care* 2006; **17**: 255–262.

DeVita MA, Groeger J, Truog R. Current controversies in critical care ethics: not just end of life. *Crit Care Med* 2003; **31** (5 Suppl.): S343.

Frenkel M. Refusing treatment. *The Oncologist* 2013; **18**: 634–636.

General Medical Council *Treatment and Care Towards the End of Life*. London: GMC Publishing; 2010.

General Medical Council. *Good Clinical Practice*; London: GMC; 2013.

Leadership Alliance for the Care of Dying People (2014) *One Chance to get it Right*. Available online: https://www.gov.uk/government/uploads/system/uploads/attachment_data/file/323188/One_chance_to_get_it_right.pdf

Relevant articles from the European Convention on Human Rights

- **Article 2**: with the exception of the prevention of criminal acts or lawful use of the death penalty, everyone's right to life shall be protected.

- **Article 3**: no one shall be subjected to torture or inhuman or degrading treatment or punishment.

- **Article 8**: within the norms of a democratic society an organisation cannot interfere with the rights of an individual unless it is to uphold the law or protect the rights and freedoms of others.

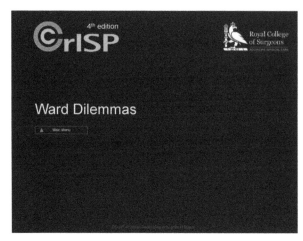

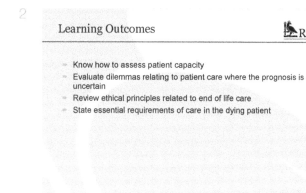

Learning Outcomes RCS

- Know how to assess patient capacity
- Evaluate dilemmas relating to patient care where the prognosis is uncertain
- Review ethical principles related to end of life care
- State essential requirements of care in the dying patient

Scenario One RCS

- You've been called by the O and G senior trainee to review a 58-year-old woman with abdominal pain.
- She has been in hospital for 4-days undergoing "potentially curative" chemotherapy for recurrent ovarian cancer.
- She has been feeling generally unwell with nausea for 36-hours
- She is on 4-hourly obs with a NEWS of 3 and just returned from the radiology department after a CT scan.

What would you do?

Managing the critically ill surgical patient RCS

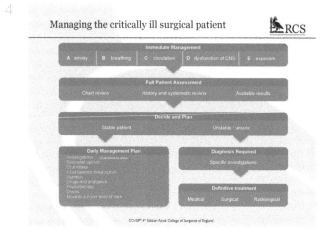

Scenario One: initial assessment RCS

A Clear but weak cough
B RR 37/min
    SaO$_2$ 98% (4l/min)
C HR 147/min, regular
    BP 114/48
    CRT 4 secs
    Urine <30ml/hour
D AVPU   Voice
E Temp.   37.2°C

Total NEWS score = 14

Immediate Management RCS

- Oxygen: increased to 15l/minute
- Fluid Challenge of 1000ml of Hartmann's solution
- Investigations already performed:
  - Haematology: FBC and coagulation studies
  - Biochemistry: U and E, LFT, Mg^{2+}, Ca^{2+}, Glucose, arterial blood gases
  - CXR, AXR, abdominal & thoracic CT with contrast

Notes Review RCS

- Salpingo-oopherectomy 3 years ago for stage 2a ovarian cancer
- Chemotherapy pre and post-operatively
- GP admission 4 days earlier with pelvic pain and iron-deficiency anaemia
- CT: pelvic mass (recurrence)
- "Potentially curative" chemotherapy commenced

Obs Chart Review RCS

- Minimal improvement since admission to hospital
- Worse in previous 36-hours
  - Loss of appetite
  - Nausea
  - Vomiting
  - Abdominal pain
  - Drowsiness

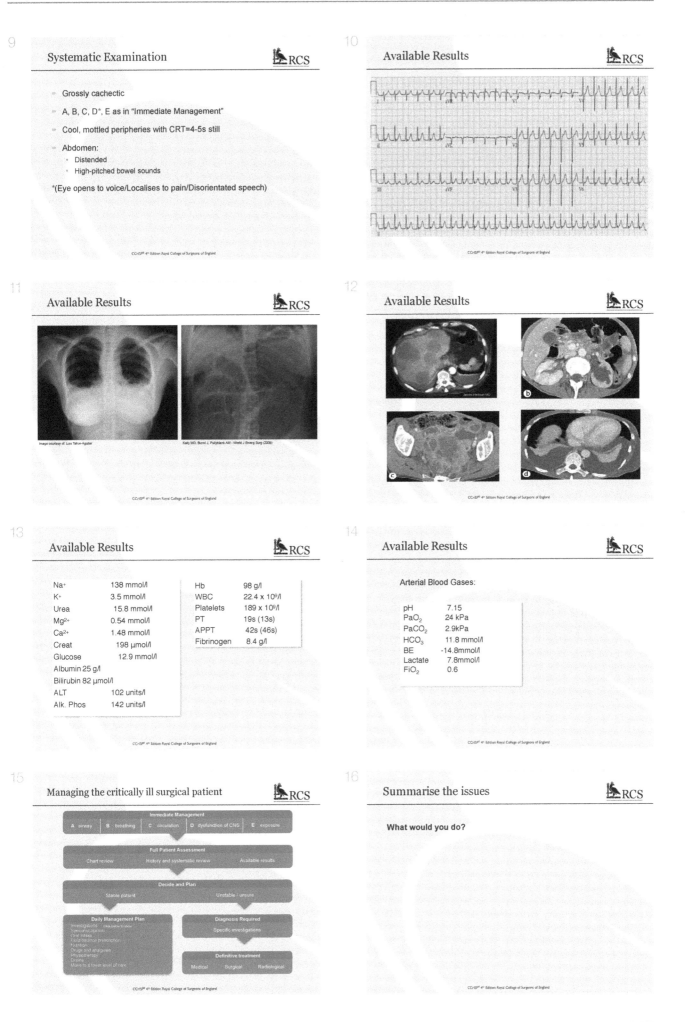

9 Systematic Examination — RCS

- Grossly cachectic
- A, B, C, D*, E as in "Immediate Management"
- Cool, mottled peripheries with CRT=4-5s still
- Abdomen:
  - Distended
  - High-pitched bowel sounds

*(Eye opens to voice/Localises to pain/Disorientated speech)

10 Available Results — RCS

11 Available Results — RCS

12 Available Results — RCS

13 Available Results — RCS

Na+	138 mmol/l	Hb	98 g/l
K+	3.5 mmol/l	WBC	22.4 x 10⁹/l
Urea	15.8 mmol/l	Platelets	189 x 10⁹/l
Mg2+	0.54 mmol/l	PT	19s (13s)
Ca2+	1.48 mmol/l	APPT	42s (46s)
Creat	198 µmol/l	Fibrinogen	8.4 g/l
Glucose	12.9 mmol/l		
Albumin 25 g/l			
Bilirubin 82 µmol/l			
ALT	102 units/l		
Alk. Phos	142 units/l		

14 Available Results — RCS

Arterial Blood Gases:

pH	7.15
PaO₂	24 kPa
PaCO₂	2.9kPa
HCO₃	11.8 mmol/l
BE	-14.8mmol/l
Lactate	7.8mmol/l
FiO₂	0.6

15 Managing the critically ill surgical patient — RCS

16 Summarise the issues — RCS

What would you do?

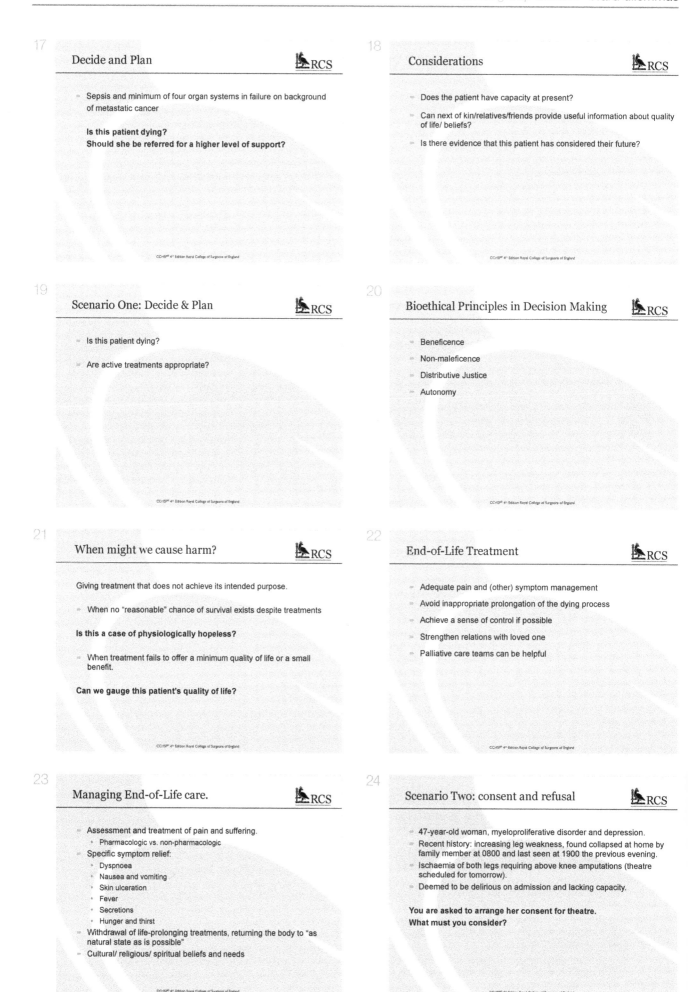

17

Decide and Plan   RCS

- Sepsis and minimum of four organ systems in failure on background of metastatic cancer

Is this patient dying?
Should she be referred for a higher level of support?

18

Considerations   RCS

- Does the patient have capacity at present?
- Can next of kin/relatives/friends provide useful information about quality of life/ beliefs?
- Is there evidence that this patient has considered their future?

19

Scenario One: Decide & Plan   RCS

- Is this patient dying?
- Are active treatments appropriate?

20

Bioethical Principles in Decision Making   RCS

- Beneficence
- Non-maleficence
- Distributive Justice
- Autonomy

21

When might we cause harm?   RCS

Giving treatment that does not achieve its intended purpose.

- When no "reasonable" chance of survival exists despite treatments

Is this a case of physiologically hopeless?

- When treatment fails to offer a minimum quality of life or a small benefit.

Can we gauge this patient's quality of life?

22

End-of-Life Treatment   RCS

- Adequate pain and (other) symptom management
- Avoid inappropriate prolongation of the dying process
- Achieve a sense of control if possible
- Strengthen relations with loved one
- Palliative care teams can be helpful

23

Managing End-of-Life care.   RCS

- Assessment and treatment of pain and suffering.
  - Pharmacologic vs. non-pharmacologic
- Specific symptom relief:
  - Dyspnoea
  - Nausea and vomiting
  - Skin ulceration
  - Fever
  - Secretions
  - Hunger and thirst
- Withdrawal of life-prolonging treatments, returning the body to "as natural state as is possible"
- Cultural/ religious/ spiritual beliefs and needs

24

Scenario Two: consent and refusal   RCS

- 47-year-old woman, myeloproliferative disorder and depression.
- Recent history: increasing leg weakness, found collapsed at home by family member at 0800 and last seen at 1900 the previous evening.
- Ischaemia of both legs requiring above knee amputations (theatre scheduled for tomorrow).
- Deemed to be delirious on admission and lacking capacity.

You are asked to arrange her consent for theatre.
What must you consider?

25

The Doctrine of Double Effect. RCS

"not forbidden to bring about a 'bad' result if the result is foreseen but not intended."

A risk-benefit assessment:
- The action has a good element.
- The intent is solely to produce the good effect.
- There is sufficient reason to permit the bad effect.
- The good effect is not achieved through the bad effect.

26

Scenario Two: capacity RCS

- Understand relevant information?
- Retain that information?
- Use that information in decision making?
- Communicate their decision?

27

Scenario Two: consent and refusal RCS

Day Two:

- Able to retain information and convinced intensivist, surgeon, anaesthetist and psychiatrist that she had capacity
- Refused surgery and stated that she was aware of consequences

What next?

28

Scenario Two RCS

- Consider your management if patient consents to surgery
- Consider your management if patient refuses treatment
- Would you set up a DNACPR order?

29

"Informed refusal" RCS

GMC: Good Medical Practice

"You must respect a competent patient's decision to refuse an investigation or treatment, even if you think their decision is wrong or irrational. You may advise the patient of your clinical opinion, but you must not put pressure on them to accept your advice. You must be careful that your words and actions do not imply judgment of the patient or their beliefs and values."

30

RCS

Any questions?

31

Summary RCS

- Surgical ward dilemmas are complex and frequently subjective
- Surgery/escalations of care may not always the best option for a patient
- Dying patients need to be recognised and actively managed
- An ethical framework and should be used for decision-making in surgical care
- Good communication and planning is needed to manage expectations

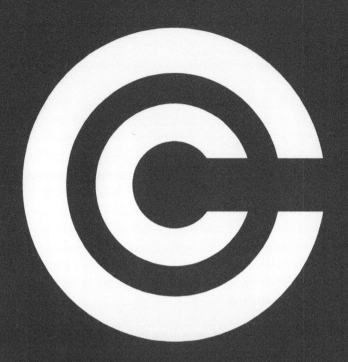

2.2

Small group session
Pain management

Introduction

This session explains the importance of pain and effective analgesia in the surgical patient. It covers the central role of the surgical trainee in the management of perioperative or post-traumatic pain, in the recognition of complications of various analgesic regimens/techniques, the recognition of when escalating pain is secondary to a surgical complication and recognition of when to refer a surgical patient to the acute pain team will be discussed.

Duration	45 minutes
Style	Small group teaching with interactive discussion
Faculty	One or two with at least one with anaesthetic knowledge and skills
AV	PowerPoint presentation

Materials

▶ 2.2.0 Patient on PCA.

▶ 2.2.1 Analgesia ladder.

Learning outcomes

At the end of this session, participants will be able to:

- understand that poor pain control can result in complications after surgery, particularly respiratory complications, and is bad for the patient;

- recognise that surgical complications may be the cause of worsening pain control;

- describe the effect of pain or analgesia on immediate patient assessment;

- evaluate multiple modes of analgesia to improve pain control while maintaining a low toxicity profile.

Teaching outline

This is an interactive session based on two scenarios.

After the objectives slide, **slides 3** and **4** outline the link between poor pain management and the development of surgical complications with poorer outcomes for patients. **Slide 4** outlines the strategies to reduce pain.

Each scenario should take 15 minutes.

Scenario 1 (**slides 5–20**) is a patient who has pain after cholecystectomy. This case introduces the links between surgical complications as a cause of poor pain control and the use of an analgesic ladder to allow consideration of routes and types of analgesia.

In this case it is worth noting the following:

- Oral agents need to be given regularly and in adequate doses in patients who have a functioning gastrointestinal tract.

- IV bolus therapy is rapid but patients receiving infusions need close monitoring owing to the potential for drug accumulation.

- PCA is safe and often effective in conscious patients but it is not suitable for all patients.

- IM therapy is now seldom used.

Scenario 2 (**slides 21–31**) is a patient who has apparently simple rib fractures that lead to a life-threatening complication of haemothorax. After successful resuscitation and management of the rib fractures and bleeding, consideration needs to be given to the need to provide effective analgesia.

In this case it is worth noting the following points:

- Epidural infusions can be very effective but they can cause hypotension and the patient requires careful monitoring.

- Other adjuvant therapies (ketamine, gabapentin, etc) are used in more complex analgesic regimens.

Slide 31 deals with the management of perioperative nausea and vomiting.

Slide 33 provides the summary key points linking back to the session objectives.

Timeline

Introduction and objectives	3 mins
Outlining link between surgical causes of pain and importance of analgesia	5 mins
Scenario 1	16 mins
Scenario 2	16 mins
Questions and summary	5 mins

1

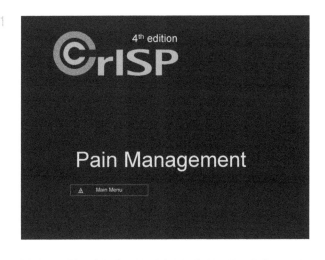

4th edition

CrISP

Pain Management

⚠ Main Menu

2

Learning Outcomes RCS

- Outline your role in the management of acute pain throughout the continuum of surgical care
- Adopt the practical and decision making skills necessary to manage pain
- Evaluate the complications from use of analgesics and analgesic techniques
- Operate as a member of a multi-disciplinary pain team

CCrISP® 4th Edition Royal College of Surgeons of England

3

What are the consequences of pain? RCS

- Mostly harmful:
  - suffering
  - impaired mobility / increased thromboembolic events
  - impaired **ventilation**
  - ↑ adrenergic surge: heart rate and vasoconstriction
  - nausea
  - hyperglycaemia
  - increased metabolic rate and catabolism
  - retention of fluids and fluid shifts

CCrISP® 4th Edition Royal College of Surgeons of England

4

Different strategies to reduce pain

- Eliminate cause
- Attenuate local inflammatory responses
- Block nerve transmission
- Modify central perception / processing

For any method we need to balance efficacy against s

5

Scenario One RCS

- You are called to see a 45 year old woman, smokes 30cpd, 1 day after laparoscopic converted to open cholecystectomy
- Distressed, says she can't move
- Short of breath, febrile

How do you assess her and what are the relevant issues regarding her pain and pain control?

CCrISP® 4th Edition Royal College of Surgeons of England

6

Acute pain management RCS

- You are contacted about a post-op patient developing worsening pain, **you must establish what the cause of worsening pain is.**

- Causes:
  - the development of a surgical complication
  - poor choice of method of pain relief
  - incorrect implementation of the chosen method

CCrISP® 4th Edition Royal College of Surgeons of England

7

Surgical causes of pain RCS

- Wounds
- Leaks
- Obstruction
- Collections
- Compartment syndrome
- Dehiscence
- Infection

CCrISP® 4th Edition Royal College of Surgeons of England

8

RCS

| Immediate Management | | | | |
| A airway | B breathing | C circulation | D dysfunction of CNS | E exposure |

| Full Patient Assessment | | |
| Chart review | History and systematic review | Available results |

| Decide and Plan | |
| Stable patient | Unstable / unsure |

| Daily Management Plan | Diagnosis Required |
| Investigations   Click below to show Specialist opinion Oral intake Fluid balance prescription Nutrition Drugs and analgesia Physiotherapy Drains Move to a lower level of care | Specific investigations |

| | Definitive treatment | | |
| | Medical | Surgical | Radiological |

CCrISP® 4th Edition Royal College of Surgeons of England

9

Scenario One
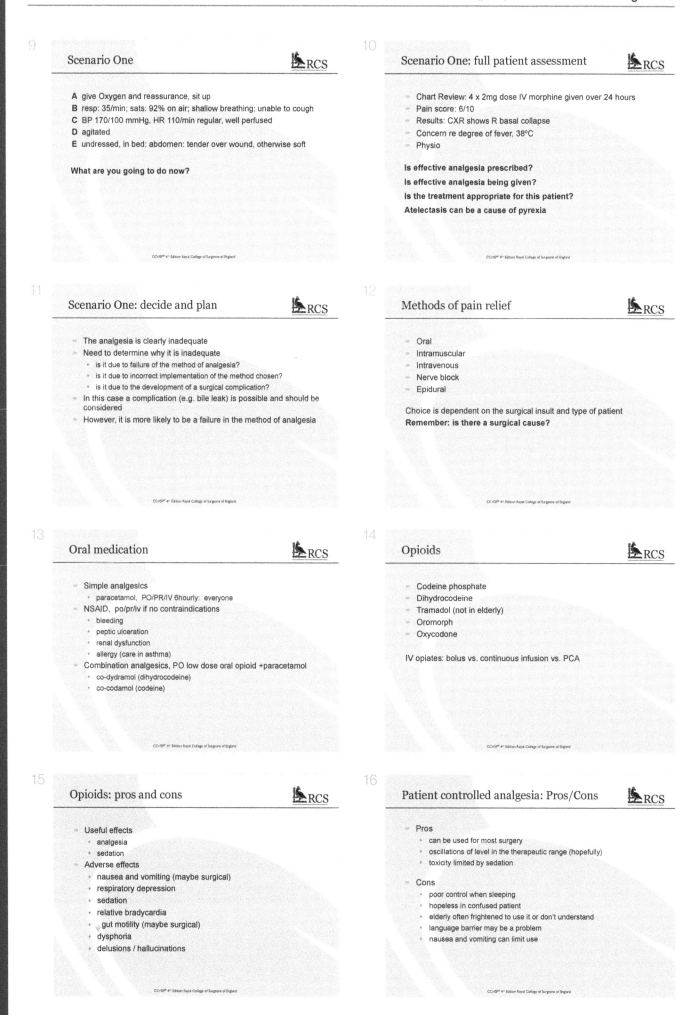

A give Oxygen and reassurance, sit up
B resp: 35/min; sats: 92% on air; shallow breathing; unable to cough
C BP 170/100 mmHg, HR 110/min regular, well perfused
D agitated
E undressed, in bed: abdomen: tender over wound, otherwise soft

What are you going to do now?

10

Scenario One: full patient assessment

- Chart Review: 4 x 2mg dose IV morphine given over 24 hours
- Pain score: 6/10
- Results: CXR shows R basal collapse
- Concern re degree of fever, 38°C
- Physio

Is effective analgesia prescribed?
Is effective analgesia being given?
Is the treatment appropriate for this patient?
Atelectasis can be a cause of pyrexia

11

Scenario One: decide and plan

- The analgesia is clearly inadequate
- Need to determine why it is inadequate
  - is it due to failure of the method of analgesia?
  - is it due to incorrect implementation of the method chosen?
  - is it due to the development of a surgical complication?
- In this case a complication (e.g. bile leak) is possible and should be considered
- However, it is more likely to be a failure in the method of analgesia

12

Methods of pain relief

- Oral
- Intramuscular
- Intravenous
- Nerve block
- Epidural

Choice is dependent on the surgical insult and type of patient
Remember: is there a surgical cause?

13

Oral medication

- Simple analgesics
  - paracetamol, PO/PR/IV 6hourly: everyone
- NSAID, po/pr/iv if no contraindications
  - bleeding
  - peptic ulceration
  - renal dysfunction
  - allergy (care in asthma)
- Combination analgesics, PO low dose oral opioid +paracetamol
  - co-dydramol (dihydrocodeine)
  - co-codamol (codeine)

14

Opioids

- Codeine phosphate
- Dihydrocodeine
- Tramadol (not in elderly)
- Oromorph
- Oxycodone

IV opiates: bolus vs. continuous infusion vs. PCA

15

Opioids: pros and cons

- Useful effects
  - analgesia
  - sedation
- Adverse effects
  - nausea and vomiting (maybe surgical)
  - respiratory depression
  - sedation
  - relative bradycardia
  - gut motility (maybe surgical)
  - dysphoria
  - delusions / hallucinations

16

Patient controlled analgesia: Pros/Cons

- Pros
  - can be used for most surgery
  - oscillations of level in the therapeutic range (hopefully)
  - toxicity limited by sedation
- Cons
  - poor control when sleeping
  - hopeless in confused patient
  - elderly often frightened to use it or don't understand
  - language barrier may be a problem
  - nausea and vomiting can limit use

17

Local anaesthetic nerve blocks/infusions RCS

- Local anaesthetic drug infusion
  - local to the wound
  - femoral nerve
  - upper and lower limb plexus
  - Interpleural / paravertebral
- Drug toxicity: rare because low concentration (0.1%) used
- May need additional pain relief
- May mask neurological signs (compartment syndrome)

CCrISP® 4ᵗʰ Edition Royal College of Surgeons of England

18

Multimodal therapy RCS

- Giving maximal analgesia with minimal side effects
- This means combinations of drugs and/or using different routes of administration, for example
  - epidural and NSAID / paracetamol
  - PCA and paracetamol / NSAID / weak opiates
- The analgesic ladder

CCrISP® 4ᵗʰ Edition Royal College of Surgeons of England

19

The analgesic ladder RCS

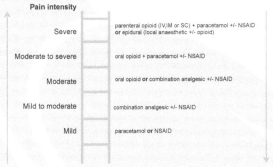

Pain intensity	
Severe	parenteral opioid (IV,IM or SC) + paracetamol +/- NSAID or epidural (local anaesthetic +/- opioid)
Moderate to severe	oral opioid + paracetamol +/- NSAID
Moderate	oral opioid **or** combination analgesic +/- NSAID
Mild to moderate	combination analgesic +/- NSAID
Mild	paracetamol **or** NSAID

CCrISP® 4ᵗʰ Edition Royal College of Surgeons of England

20

Scenario One: plan RCS

- Rule out a major surgical complication
  - ultrasound or CT abdomen?
- Titrate morphine dose until analgesia is achieved
- Add other modes (e.g. regular background oral or rectal paracetamol and a NSAID)
- Consider PCA

CCrISP® 4ᵗʰ Edition Royal College of Surgeons of England

21

Scenario Two RCS

- 79 year old independently living man; fell from one step onto left hand side. Fractured left 3-7 ribs, no other injuries. In Emergency Medicine dept.:
  - A Speaking clearly, in pain
  - B RR 18/min, shallow breaths
  - C BP 170/96 mmHg, HR 106/min, regular
  - D Orientated, in pain, distressed
  - E Bruised left chest

How are you going to manage this patient?

What complications will you anticipate?

CCrISP® 4ᵗʰ Edition Royal College of Surgeons of England

22

Scenario Two: ward management RCS

- Admitted to surgical ward:
  - Humidified oxygen
  - Paracetamol
  - Gabapentin
  - Oxycodone PCA or epidural
  - Regular lactulose
  - CXR

CCrISP® 4ᵗʰ Edition Royal College of Surgeons of England

23

24

Scenario Two – 36 hours later RCS

- You are called to the ward: patient is peri-arrest
  - A Grunting, snoring sound
  - B RR 28/min, poor AE, sats: 90%
  - C BP 70/45 mmHg, HR 120/min (reg), sweaty & clammy
  - D Unresponsive
  - E In bed

What is your differential diagnosis?

How are you going to manage this patient?

CCrISP® 4ᵗʰ Edition Royal College of Surgeons of England

25

Scenario Two: decide and plan

How are you going to manage this patient?

- Give oxygen
- 1L crystalloid stat (a further 2L given over next 60 mins)
- Hb 54 g/L (previously 137 g/L)
- Lactate 9.8 mmol/L
- Portable CXR

26

27

Scenario Two: decide and plan

- Admitted to ICU and intubated and ventilated
- Transfused 4 units of blood
- CT chest: large left haemothorax
- Ribs were internally reduced and stabilised and haemothorax was drained.
- Epidural at T4: 0.1% bupivacaine + fentanyl 2mcg/ml
- Once epidural established -- weaned off ventilation
- Next day T/F to HDU, where he was converted to fentanyl PCA, paracetamol and regular ondansetron

28

Epidurals

- Indications
  - major abdominal or thoracic surgery
  - lower limb surgery
  - respiratory compromised patient
- Local anaesthetic and opiate infusion
- Bupivacaine 0.1% + fentanyl 2mcg/ml

29

Epidurals: problems

- Hypotension
- Ascending block (resp. muscle impairment)
  - stop immediately
  - assist ventilation
  - do not tilt head down
- Urinary retention without catheter
- Motor blockade: immobility pressure complications
- Side effects of opioids
- Epidural haematoma – rare but...

30

Assessing hypotension with an epidural

What is the cause?
- Vasodilation from the epidural block
- Hypovolaemia / surgical cause
- Cardiogenic shock
- Accurate diagnosis requires meticulous assessment of venous volume and adequacy of perfusion

31

Nausea and vomiting

- Can be a side effect of analgesia, but..
- Remember to look for a surgical cause, especially in scenario with worsening pain.
- Treatment
  - Metoclopromide and / or cyclizine
  - Ondansetron
  - Prochlorperazine
  - Dexamethasone
- Remember hydration and fluid balance

32

Any questions?

33

Summary

RCS

- Surgical complications may be the cause of pain
- Poor pain relief causes complications, particularly respiratory
- The effect of pain, or analgesia used to treat it, may impact on the immediate assessment
- A structured use of multiple modes of treatment is best
  - oral agents need to be regular and in adequate dose
  - IV bolus therapy is rapid but infusion needs close monitoring to keep in therapeutic range
  - PCA is safe and often effective in an awake patient but some patients are not suitable
  - epidural Infusion can be very effective but patients need careful monitoring
  - IM therapy is now seldom used

CCrISP® 4th Edition Royal College of Surgeons of England

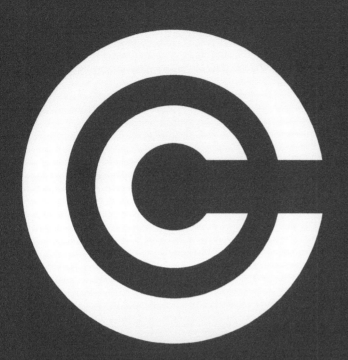

2.3

Small group session
**Respiratory care and chest
imaging**

Introduction

This session allows candidates to consider the role of radiological investigations (particularly chest imaging) in managing the major life-threatening postoperative complications of pulmonary embolism, infection and adult respiratory distress syndrome (ARDS). It links to the session on respiratory failure (1.7) and emphasises the importance of the use of the comprehensive CCrSP three-stage patient assessment, allied to proactive management of complications as they occur so that patients do not deteriorate further.

Although the session includes radiological images and ensures that candidates have a reliable system for interpretation, it should not be focused on radiological interpretation at the expense of the key clinical messages for patient management.

Duration	45 minutes
Style	Small group teaching with interactive discussion
Faculty	One or two including at least one with anaesthetic skills
AV	PowerPoint presentation

Resources

▶ CCrISP system of assessment poster.

Learning outcomes

By the end of this session, participants should be able to:

- state the key considerations for managing pulmonary embolism, infection and respiratory failure in surgical patients;

- use a system for interpreting chest radiographs;

- evaluate when to supplement the CCrISP three-stage assessment with radiological investigations;

- discuss the role of radiological imaging with physiotherapy and of additional respiratory support driving postoperative surgical patient care.

Teaching outline

This is an interactive session based on two cases.

After the objectives slide, **slides 3** and **4** provide revision on the structures that can be identified in a plain chest X-ray image and outline some simple systems that are commonly used when reviewing chest images to ensure that important pathology is not missed. **Slides 8–18** deal with the case of a patient undergoing elective total hip replacement who suffers a postoperative pulmonary embolism and subsequently develops infection in infarcted segments of lung.

Slides 19–28 relate to a patient who undergoes semiurgent ERCP for obstructive jaundice and develops post-procedure pancreatitis and respiratory failure owing to a combination of developing ARDS and pleural effusions.

Teaching outline

Slide 3 is a plain chest X-ray film. Ask candidates to describe the structures that can be seen on the film and explain the system they use to ensure they review the film systematically.

It can be helpful to ask all the candidates if they use a system and to identify what system each candidate uses (**slide 4**).

This identifies anatomical structures that can be reviewed. It is worth encouraging the candidates to discuss what pathologies might be associated with changes in the structures, eg loss of clear right heart border in right middle lobe consolidation, misplacement of trachea in a rotated film, lung collapse or pneumothorax.

Scenario 1

Slides 5–19

These slides introduce the first case and allow candidates to consider in which types of patients preoperative chest radiography should be performed. **Slide 7** refers to NICE guidance, but please make reference to the relevant guidance that applies in your territory/country. Ask the candidates to identify the patients/procedures they would consider need chest radiography.

Identify from the group whether they would have expected the patient in this scenario to have had a preoperative chest X-ray. Note that in many cancer patients undergoing surgery staging chest CT will already have been performed, obviating the need for plain chest X-rays.

Slide 7

This the same patient 4 days after her elective surgery.

Ask candidates to identify the concerning elements of the initial patient assessment and to confirm that they would treat the patient with increased oxygen. Discuss the merits of administering a fluid bolus at this point (there are arguments for and against).

Slide 8

Use this slide to prompt candidates to identify what they would pay particular attention to in the full patient assessment stage.

Slide 10

This slide should lead to discussion that a chest X-ray is now warranted as there is no obvious clinical and laboratory diagnosis, although at this stage the rise in WCC, urea and CRP associated with poor air entry could indicate a developing chest infection. Similarly, the swollen legs and lack of a pyrexia may point to other diagnoses.

Slide 11

This is a lower-quality mobile film and, apart from the suggestion of some right middle lobe changes indicated by the right heart border, there is little to suggest that the patient has a full-blown chest infection.

It would be reasonable at this point to consider alternative diagnoses and consider deep vein thrombosis (DVT)/pulmonary embolism (PE).

Slide 12

Discuss why CT pulmonary angiography (CTPA) is indicated for this patient and also the fact that a PE after major joint surgery requires senior involvement regarding plans for anticoagulation.

Slide 13

This slide introduces the same patient 1 week later. Encourage candidates to point out the concerning elements of the assessment again.

Slides 14–17

Candidates should be asked to point out the abnormal features eg right upper lobe changes, loss of volume on the right side and pleural effusion. Candidates should be asked to consider how they would treat this woman in light of her pre-existing likely anticoagulation and worsening respiratory function and reflect on whether at this stage continued care on the ward is appropriate. **Slide 17** illustrates some of the treatments that can be offered with physiotherapy but you should emphasise that the patient must be able to cooperate with these.

Scenario 2 (slides 20–29)

Slide 20

Case 2 is a 76-year-old man who develops vomiting 5 days after ERCP and sphincterotomy. Candidates are expected to use the CCrISP assessment system over the subsequent slides to work out that the patient has developed pancreatitis and is developing a number of organ dysfunctions.

Slide 21

This slide illustrates the value of a fluid challenge and the concern that oxygenation is marginal (saturations 95% on 15 litres of oxygen).

Slide 23

The ultrasound report indicates that ERCP was a reasonable plan. Some centres may advocate magnetic resonance cholangiopancreatography (MRCP) also, as ultrasound of the common bile duct may be inaccurate, but in this case it appears reasonable to have gone ahead.

Slide 24

This report indicates no unusual technical difficulties with the sphincterotomy that would account for the current symptoms.

Slide 25

The blood results are consistent with improvement, but not full recovery, after ERCP. Note the high amylase level, consistent with the development of pancreatitis.

Slide 26

This is the admission film, not the current one. It illustrates a small right pleural effusion (loss of costophrenic angle), which would not be unexpected in a patient admitted with acute obstructive jaundice.

Slides 27–29

This set of slides illustrates the change from previously, with extensive bilateral pleural effusions and increased air space shadowing. Participants should consider that this may indicate either pulmonary oedema or, of greater concern, the development of ARDS associated with the pancreatitis. This links into the development of type 2 respiratory failure (hypoxia and rising carbon dioxide levels) on the blood gas analysis and the need for escalation of care and critical care review and support.

Timeline

Introduction and objectives:	2 minutes
Outlining a system of chest X-ray interpretation and the structures that can be identified	5 minutes
Scenario 1	20 minutes
Scenario 2	15 minutes
Questions and summary	3 minutes

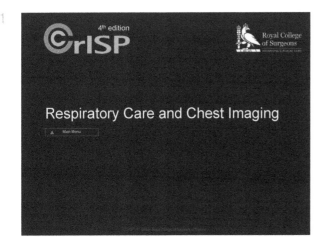

Respiratory Care and Chest Imaging

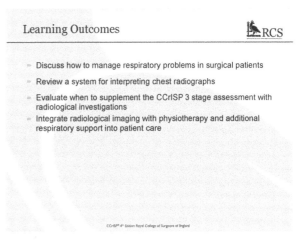

Learning Outcomes

- Discuss how to manage respiratory problems in surgical patients
- Review a system for interpreting chest radiographs
- Evaluate when to supplement the CCrISP 3 stage assessment with radiological investigations
- Integrate radiological imaging with physiotherapy and additional respiratory support into patient care

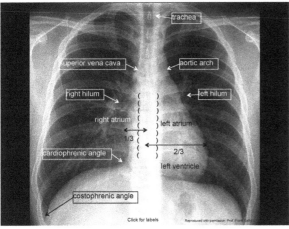

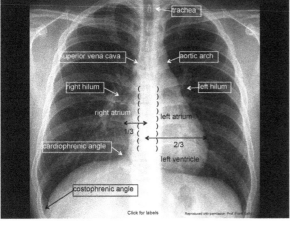

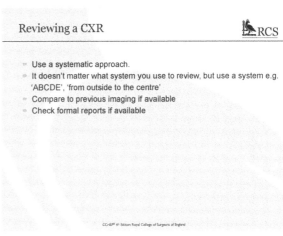

Reviewing a CXR

- Use a systematic approach.
- It doesn't matter what system you use to review, but use a system e.g. 'ABCDE', 'from outside to the centre'
- Compare to previous imaging if available
- Check formal reports if available

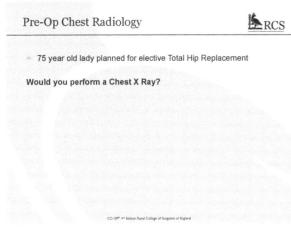

Pre-Op Chest Radiology

- 75 year old lady planned for elective Total Hip Replacement

Would you perform a Chest X Ray?

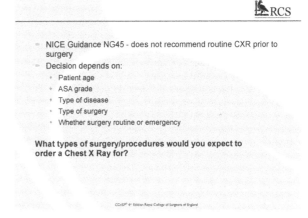

- NICE Guidance NG45 - does not recommend routine CXR prior to surgery
- Decision depends on:
  - Patient age
  - ASA grade
  - Type of disease
  - Type of surgery
  - Whether surgery routine or emergency

What types of surgery/procedures would you expect to order a Chest X Ray for?

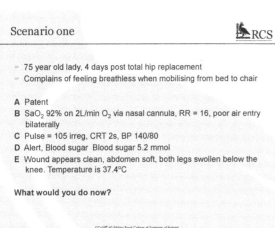

Scenario one

- 75 year old lady, 4 days post total hip replacement
- Complains of feeling breathless when mobilising from bed to chair

A Patent
B SaO$_2$ 92% on 2L/min O$_2$ via nasal cannula, RR = 16, poor air entry bilaterally
C Pulse = 105 irreg, CRT 2s, BP 140/80
D Alert, Blood sugar Blood sugar 5.2 mmol
E Wound appears clean, abdomen soft, both legs swollen below the knee. Temperature is 37.4°C

What would you do now?

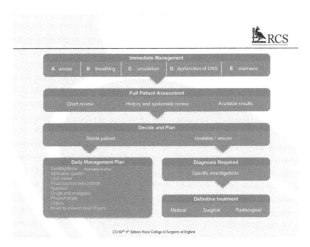

9

Full Patient Assessment

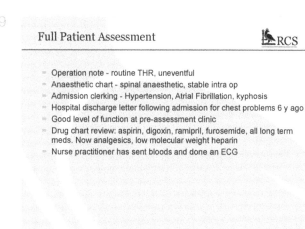

RCS

- Operation note - routine THR, uneventful
- Anaesthetic chart - spinal anaesthetic, stable intra op
- Admission clerking - Hypertension, Atrial Fibrillation, kyphosis
- Hospital discharge letter following admission for chest problems 6 y ago
- Good level of function at pre-assessment clinic
- Drug chart review: aspirin, digoxin, ramipril, furosemide, all long term meds. Now analgesics, low molecular weight heparin
- Nurse practitioner has sent bloods and done an ECG

CCrISP® 4th Edition Royal College of Surgeons of England

10

Available Results

RCS

	On admission	Today
Hb	125	133
WCC	5.4	10.6
Platelets	279	222
CRP	15	207
Na	137	130
K	4.9	5.2
Urea	5.8	10.2
Creatinine	92	106

ECG-Atrial Fibrillation, no new changes
Would you order a Chest X Ray?

CCrISP® 4th Edition Royal College of Surgeons of England

11

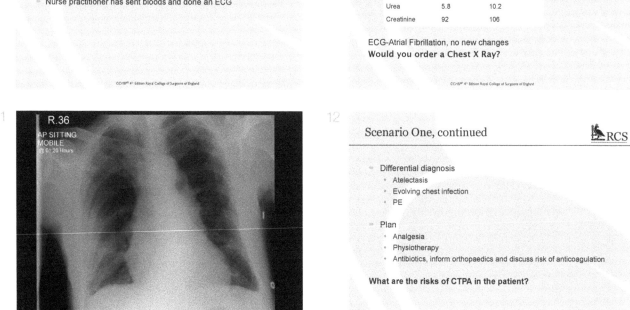

12

Scenario One, continued

RCS

- Differential diagnosis
  - Atelectasis
  - Evolving chest infection
  - PE

- Plan
  - Analgesia
  - Physiotherapy
  - Antibiotics, inform orthopaedics and discuss risk of anticoagulation

What are the risks of CTPA in the patient?

CCrISP® 4th Edition Royal College of Surgeons of England

13

Scenario One, continued

RCS

- Orthopaedics not happy with anticoagulation
- Patient worsened within 6 hours
  - HR 120/min AF
  - SpO_2 = 90% on 10L/O_2

What would you do now?

CCrISP® 4th Edition Royal College of Surgeons of England

14

What would you do next?

RCS

- Request CTPA as:
  - Patient is increasingly hypoxic
  - Worsening tachycardia
  - No response to therapy for atelectasis

CTPA report:

Extensive bilateral pulmonary emboli, with evidence of right heart strain. Small bilateral pleural effusions.

Anticoagulation after senior discussion.

CCrISP® 4th Edition Royal College of Surgeons of England

15

One week later

RCS

- You are asked to review patient again as short of breath:

A Patent
B SaO_2 92% on 15L/min O_2, RR = 30, crackles R>L
C Pulse = 115 irreg, CRT 2s, BP 90/50
D Alert, Blood sugar 5.8 mmol
E nil new

You order a CXR as part of your full patient assessment.

CCrISP® 4th Edition Royal College of Surgeons of England

16

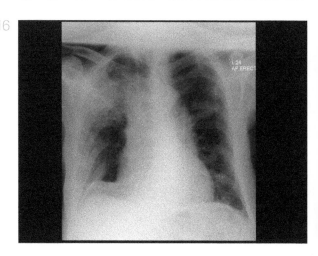

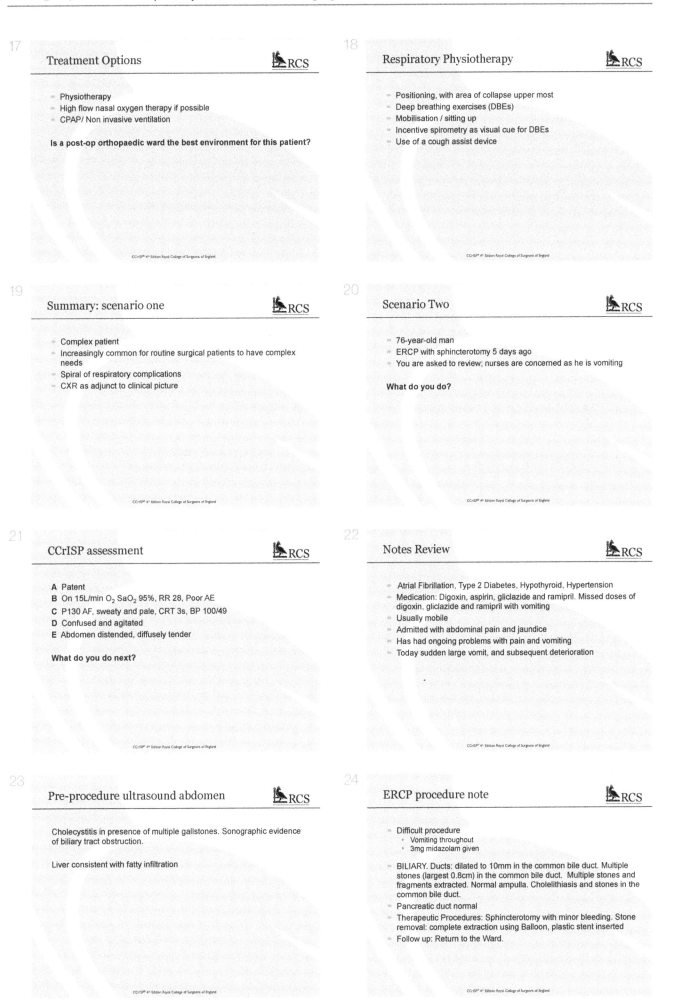

17

Treatment Options ★RCS

- Physiotherapy
- High flow nasal oxygen therapy if possible
- CPAP/ Non invasive ventilation

Is a post-op orthopaedic ward the best environment for this patient?

CCrISP® 4th Edition Royal College of Surgeons of England

18

Respiratory Physiotherapy ★RCS

- Positioning, with area of collapse upper most
- Deep breathing exercises (DBEs)
- Mobilisation / sitting up
- Incentive spirometry as visual cue for DBEs
- Use of a cough assist device

CCrISP® 4th Edition Royal College of Surgeons of England

19

Summary: scenario one ★RCS

- Complex patient
- Increasingly common for routine surgical patients to have complex needs
- Spiral of respiratory complications
- CXR as adjunct to clinical picture

CCrISP® 4th Edition Royal College of Surgeons of England

20

Scenario Two ★RCS

- 76-year-old man
- ERCP with sphincterotomy 5 days ago
- You are asked to review; nurses are concerned as he is vomiting

What do you do?

CCrISP® 4th Edition Royal College of Surgeons of England

21

CCrISP assessment ★RCS

A Patent
B On 15L/min O$_2$ SaO$_2$ 95%, RR 28, Poor AE
C P130 AF, sweaty and pale, CRT 3s, BP 100/49
D Confused and agitated
E Abdomen distended, diffusely tender

What do you do next?

CCrISP® 4th Edition Royal College of Surgeons of England

22

Notes Review ★RCS

- Atrial Fibrillation, Type 2 Diabetes, Hypothyroid, Hypertension
- Medication: Digoxin, aspirin, gliclazide and ramipril. Missed doses of digoxin, gliclazide and ramipril with vomiting
- Usually mobile
- Admitted with abdominal pain and jaundice
- Has had ongoing problems with pain and vomiting
- Today sudden large vomit, and subsequent deterioration

CCrISP® 4th Edition Royal College of Surgeons of England

23

Pre-procedure ultrasound abdomen ★RCS

Cholecystitis in presence of multiple gallstones. Sonographic evidence of biliary tract obstruction.

Liver consistent with fatty infiltration

CCrISP® 4th Edition Royal College of Surgeons of England

24

ERCP procedure note ★RCS

- Difficult procedure
  - Vomiting throughout
  - 3mg midazolam given
- BILIARY. Ducts: dilated to 10mm in the common bile duct. Multiple stones (largest 0.8cm) in the common bile duct. Multiple stones and fragments extracted. Normal ampulla. Cholelithiasis and stones in the common bile duct.
- Pancreatic duct normal
- Therapeutic Procedures: Sphincterotomy with minor bleeding. Stone removal: complete extraction using Balloon, plastic stent inserted
- Follow up: Return to the Ward.

CCrISP® 4th Edition Royal College of Surgeons of England

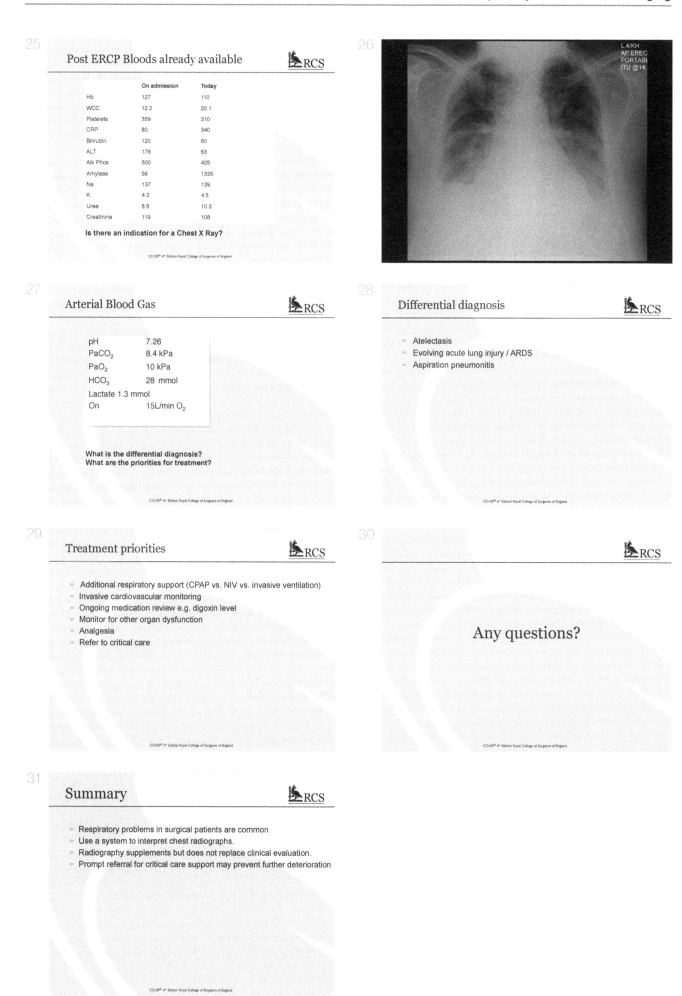

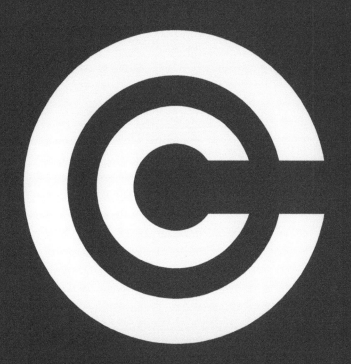

2.4

Course summary

Introduction

This session allows the course director to summarise the key messages of the course and to place them in their clinical context as the candidates begin to prepare to use their skills in their practice.

Duration	15 minutes
Style	Lecture
Faculty	One
AV	PowerPoint presentation

Objectives

- To show that the course objectives have been discussed.

- To briefly review the CCrISP system of assessment.

- To refer to the broader clinical issues on which the course touches and the breadth and limitations of the ways in which the course knowledge can be used in clinical practice.

- To discuss the mechanism and purpose of the simulated patient assessments.

Teaching outline

This lecture permits the course director to tie the course content together and relate it to the participants' clinical practice. Motivate the participants to use their new skills but also discuss the limitations of the course. The accompanying PowerPoint presentation assists in reviewing the system of assessment but clinical pictures can be used to replace or supplement this if desired.

The summary slide include the CCrISP system of assessment and the 'six As'. The six As, also known as the 'six Australian As', although coming from Australia are equally applicable in all practices.

Time may be saved during the preceding two sessions, allowing the course director to 'walk through' the simulated patient assessments, emphasising their educational (rather than confrontational) nature. Emphasise the importance of role play and of learning from the partner's performance. This should have been stressed in the faculty demonstrations earlier in the day.

Resources

▶ Laptop.

▶ Data projector.

▶ Screen.

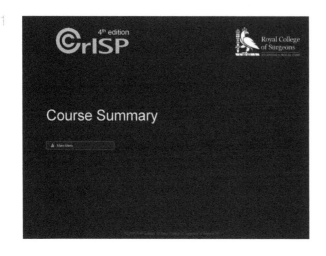

1

4th edition

CrISP

Royal College
of Surgeons

Course Summary

Main Menu

2

Course objectives

- Identify at risk patients
- Manage critically ill surgical patients:
  - marry theory to practice
  - Structured clinical assessment
- Prevent the 'complications cascade'

3

Course objectives

RCS

- Lead the ward team in surgical critical care
- Organise and communicate
  - colleagues: own specialty/other specialties
  - patients and relatives
- Assume responsibility
  - demonstrating initiative
  - being aware of limitations (others' and yours)

4

RCS

- Predict problems and act to prevent them
- Recognise when patients deteriorate
- Respond appropriately when you do

5

RCS

Immediate Management				
A airway	B breathing	C circulation	D dysfunction of CNS	E exposure

Full Patient Assessment		
Chart review	History and systematic review	Available results

Decide and Plan	
Stable patient	Unstable / unsure

Daily Management Plan
Investigations
Specialist opinion
Oral intake
Fluid balance, prescription
nutrition
Drugs and analgesia
Physiotherapy
Drains
Move to a lower level of care

Diagnosis Required
Specific investigations

Definitive treatment		
Medical	Surgical	Radiological

6

Summative Assessment

RCS

- Set up
  - 8 candidates, 4 pairs, 1 being tested, 1 observing
  - Other 8 candidates do the virtual ward round
  - Groups then swap over after a coffee break for each group
- Video demonstrating expectations of the moulage
  - Realism
  - Actively demonstrate what you can do
  - Don't jump to conclusions
  - There are no catches

7

RCS

Any questions?

8

Summary

RCS

- Accept responsibility for patient management
- Adopt a systematic approach to patient assessment
- Appreciate that complications tend to cascade rapidly
- Anticipate and prevent complications with simple, timely actions
- Apply effective communication skills to facilitate patient care
- Ask for appropriate assistance in a timely manner

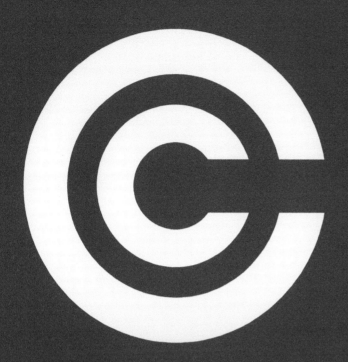

2.5

Demonstration
Practical management of the critically ill surgical patient: a faculty demonstration

This is the final lecture of the course and introduces the simulated patient testing and video demonstration of the assessment to give candidates an indication of what is expected of them. It is usually given by the course director and is an opportunity for the director to restate the CCrISP philosophy of looking after potentially sick surgical patients.

It should be interactive and give the candidates a last chance to ask questions and to clarify any outstanding issues they may have. It then goes onto explain the organisation of the final sessions of the course. There is no need to go into the detail of the three-stage assessment process as this will be covered in the video of a faculty demonstration of the final moulage.

Learning outcomes

At the end of this session, participants will be able to:

- summarise the three-stage assessment process;

- recognise the importance of accurate patient assessment;

- demonstrate the importance of recognising deteriorating patients;

- demonstrate the importance of communication to ensure that patients have the best chance of experiencing good outcomes.

Equipment

▶ Computer.

▶ PowerPoint presentation.

▶ Large screen

Timeline

This session lasts 40 minutes. There are two videos linked to the CCrISP PowerPoint, the Faculty Demonstration Patient Assessment (parts 1 and 2 of the scenario) and the Professional Skills communication session (part 3 of the scenario).

The Demonstration Assessment video is based on a patient with Crohn's disease who has emergency surgery followed by an anastomotic leak and a subsequent pulmonary embolism. This video lasts for 37 minutes but can be stopped after 20 minutes at the completion of part 1 of the scenario.

Video timings

Scenario part 1:   0 – 20 mins, including setting the scenario

Scenario part 2:   20 – 36 mins

                ECG trace shown at 29:00

                Key messages shown at 36:06

The Professional Skills video is part 3 of the scenario. This lasts for 8.5 minutes.

The course PowerPoint contains examples of the notes used in the scenario. You don't need to run the PowerPoint alongside the video: test results are given verbally and in some cases written on the screen.

The CCrISP system of assessment

Immediate management
Airway | Breathing | Circulation | Dysfunction of CNS | Exposure

Full patient assessment
Chart review | History and systematic examination | Available results

Decide and plan
Unstable/unsure   Stable

Diagnosis required
Specific investigations

Definitive treatment
Medical | Surgical | Radiological

Investigations
Blood | X-ray

Specialist opinion

Nutrition
Requirement | Route

Fluid balance prescription

Oral intake

Drugs and analgesia
Treat condition | Prophylaxis | Comorbid disease

Physiotherapy
Chest | Mobility

Drains and tubes removal

Move to a lower level of care

1

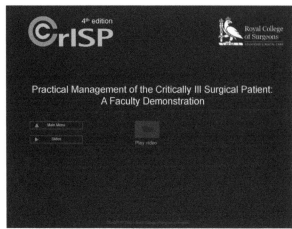

2

Objectives

- To demonstrate a 'real-time' practical management of the critically ill surgical patient
- To highlight the principles of the course and revise the CCrISP protocol
- To demonstrate teamwork and communication skills
- To introduce the final assessed practical management scenarios
- To discuss the role of feedback and appraisal

3

Brief to candidate

- It is 5pm and you are the middle grade surgeon on duty in a teaching hospital
- Your team comprises a foundation year trainee and consultant (Mr Martin Soul), who is interviewing at the University
- You have been called urgently to the surgical ward to see a 39 year old woman who has been deteriorating on the ward
- A staff nurse says the patient is complaining of worsening pain. She had a bowel operation 5 days ago
  - the nurse has taken observations which show a temperature of 39°C, RR 26/min, BP 90/60 mmHg and HR 120/min regular

4

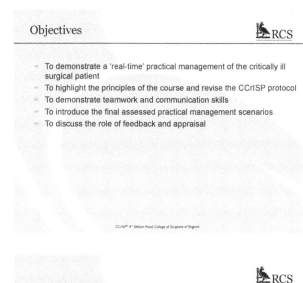

5

Immediate management: summary

- A Patent, 15l oxygen
- B SaO$_2$ 96%. Tachypneic
- C BP 90/60 mmHg, HR 120/min regular, cool, clammy
  - IV access, fluid challenge, bloods
- D In pain, distressed, BM6
- E Abdomen tender

6

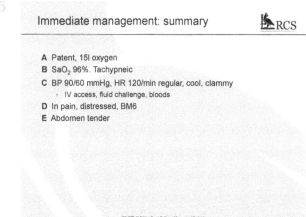

7

Notes review

- Known Crohn's disease
- Worsening diarrhoea and weight loss despite azothioprine and mesalazine
- Previous pulmonary embolus
- Now 5 days post semi-urgent subtotal colectomy/ ileo-rectal anastomosis: difficult but no stoma
- Slow progress with pain/poor mobilisation, spiking temps
- Taking sips, minimal passed PR

8

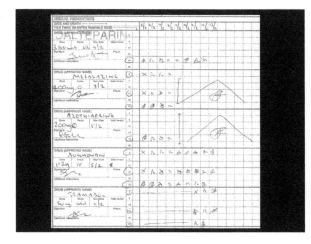

9

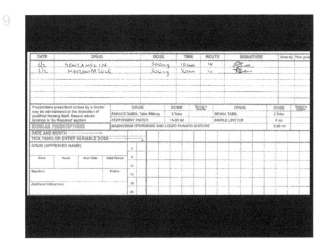

10

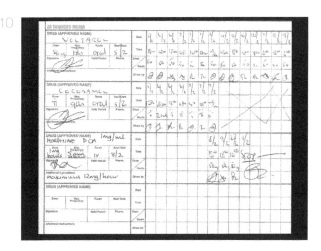

11

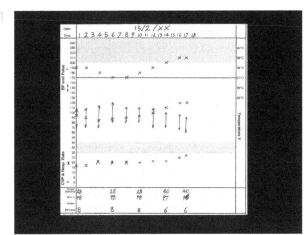

12

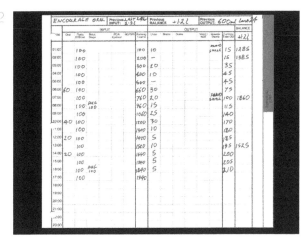

13

Available results

RCS

Hb	8.6 g/dl	ABG	(FiO$_2$:1)
WCC	18 x10^9/l	pH	7.36
Platelets	102 x10^9/l	PaO$_2$	20.4 kPa
Urea	8.1 mmol/l	PaCO$_2$	4.1 kPa
Creatinine	93 μmol/l	HCO$_3$	17 mmol/l
K	3.2 mmol/l	BE	-6
Na	134 mmol/l	Lactate	3 mmol/l
Clotting	INR 1.1		

CCrISP® 4th Edition Royal College of Surgeons of England

14

Previous results

RCS

	5/2	9/2	11/2
Hb	9.6	8.8	8.9
WCC	16	19	17
Platelet	145	138	122
INR	1.0	1.0	1.1
Na	139	136	134
K	5.1	4.5	3.6
Cl	101	103	104
Urea	6.3	7.1	7.4
Creatinine	56	88	75
Mg			0.65
Phosphate			0.68

CCrISP® 4th Edition Royal College of Surgeons of England

15

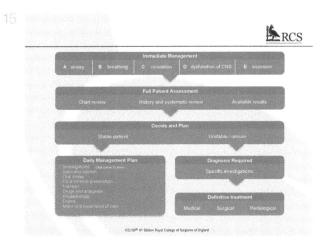

16

Decide and plan

RCS

Unstable
- Continue resuscitation
  - oxygen
  - IV fluid
  - higher level of care
- Investigations
  - CT scan
  - CXR
- Communicate
  - HDU
  - Consultant
  - patient/relatives

CCrISP® 4th Edition Royal College of Surgeons of England

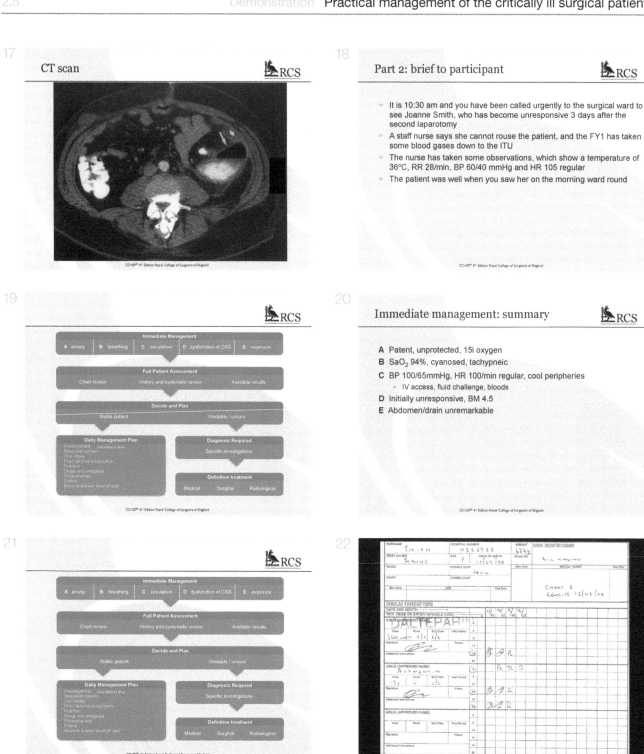

17

CT scan   ♜RCS

18

Part 2: brief to participant   ♜RCS

- It is 10:30 am and you have been called urgently to the surgical ward to see Joanne Smith, who has become unresponsive 3 days after the second laparotomy
- A staff nurse says she cannot rouse the patient, and the FY1 has taken some blood gases down to the ITU
- The nurse has taken some observations, which show a temperature of 36°C, RR 28/min, BP 60/40 mmHg and HR 105 regular
- The patient was well when you saw her on the morning ward round

19

♜RCS

20

Immediate management: summary   ♜RCS

- **A** Patent, unprotected, 15l oxygen
- **B** SaO$_2$ 94%, cyanosed, tachypneic
- **C** BP 100/65mmHg, HR 100/min regular, cool peripheries
  - IV access, fluid challenge, bloods
- **D** Initially unresponsive, BM 4.5
- **E** Abdomen/drain unremarkable

21

♜RCS

22

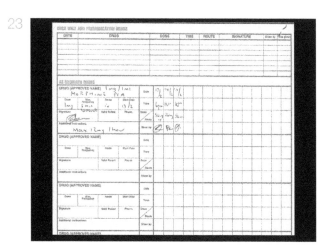

23

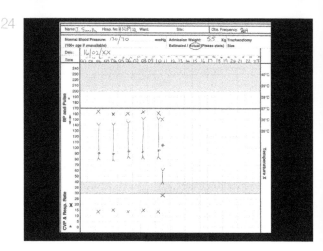

24

25

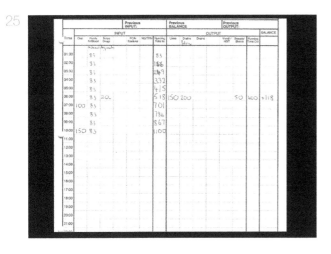

26

Available results

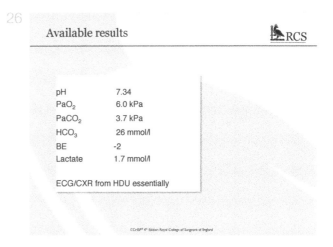

pH	7.34
PaO$_2$	6.0 kPa
PaCO$_2$	3.7 kPa
HCO$_3$	26 mmol/l
BE	-2
Lactate	1.7 mmol/l

ECG/CXR from HDU essentially

27

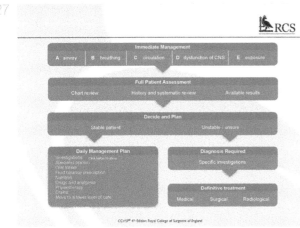

28

Investigations

Hb	8.8 g/dl
WCC	11.7 x10^9/l
Platelets	180 x10^9/l
Urea	6.1 mmol/l
Creatinine	93 μmol/l
K	3.6 mmol/l
Na	138 mmol/l
Clotting INR 1.1	

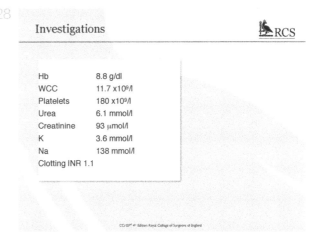

29

ABG

	On air	FiO$_2$: 1
pH7.34	7.36	
PaO$_2$	6.0 kPa	10.8 kPa
PaCO$_2$	3.7 kPa	3.2 kPa
HCO$_3$	26 mmol/l	26 mmol/l
BE	-2	-1
Lactate	1.7 mmol/l	1.2 mmol/l

30

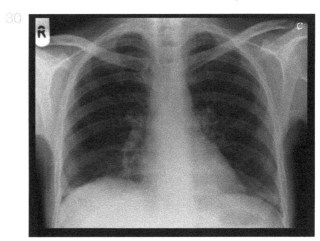

31

ECG

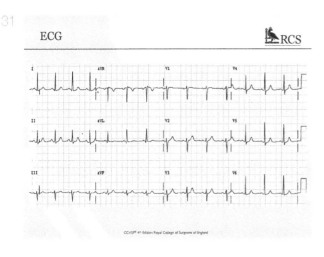

32

Plan of action 1

- Continue high flow oxygen/monitoring
- CT Angiogram
- Doppler leg veins
- Heparinisation
- Lysis?
- Cultures
- US/CT abdo?

33

Radiology report

- On duplex ultrasound, the left popliteal vein is non compressible. The appearance is suggestive of thrombus. The femoral and iliac vein demonstrate normal flow with no evidence of extension of thrombus. Normal examination on the right
- CT pulmonary angiogram: bilateral areas of malperfusion are identified. The appearances are highly suggestive of acute pulmonary emboli

34

Plan of action 2

- Communication with
  - HDU
  - senior colleagues
  - patient and relatives
  - nursing staff
  - physiotherapists
- Documentation

35

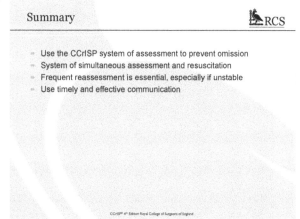

36

Any questions?

37

Summary

- Use the CCrISP system of assessment to prevent omission
- System of simultaneous assessment and resuscitation
- Frequent reassessment is essential, especially if unstable
- Use timely and effective communication

38

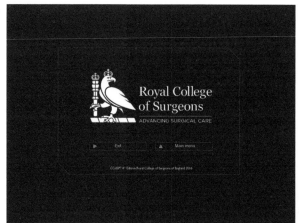

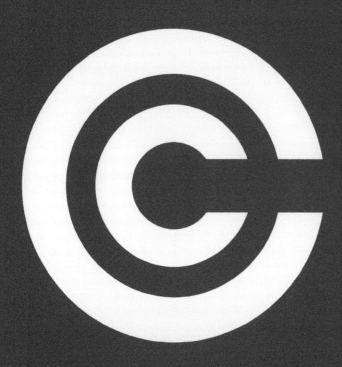

Practical session
Moulage instructions

Introduction

In this session the participants will manage a simulated patient according to the CCrISP system. This involves assessment, interpretation of results, decision-making, planning and communication.

Duration	180 minutes (four 45-minute rotations)
Style	Practical
Faculty	Eight
AV	NA

Objectives

- To allow each participant to manage a simulated critically ill patient and indicate if he or she can integrate course material into clinical practice.

- To enable each candidate to evaluate a colleague's performance and to learn from observation.

- To indicate where course material fits in to 'real' practice.

- To assess each participant's performance.

- To permit faculty to reinforce any identified weak areas.

Teaching outline

The simulated patient case scenarios can be stressful for candidates but they should be used to encourage them to demonstrate their abilities. The aim of the scenarios is to offer candidates the chance to use some of their new skills in a realistic environment under a degree of pressure and with the opportunity for immediate feedback and discussion. The scenarios also provide an opportunity for the instructors to assess the participants' performance, with some opportunity for immediate learning and reinforcement.

There are four simulated patient stations with two faculty at each – ideally a surgeon and a non-surgeon should be paired. Faculty stay with the same patient and run the scenario four times. Participants rotate in pairs – one participant manages the first patient for 45 minutes while the partner watches and gives feedback. They then move on to another patient (and a different scenario) and reverse roles. On most courses, the course director selects two scenarios to use (there are three scenarios to choose from), so there are effectively two pairs of stations. It is important that the faculty teach on their appointed station and that candidates rotate correctly, otherwise they might see the same patient scenario twice.

The cases are based on situations encountered with real surgical patients. The scenarios cover three episodes and are therefore quite complex. Instructors are provided with a written script, together with case notes, investigations and radiographs. The documentation will ease the task facing you but planning beforehand is essential. You will need to familiarise yourself with the scenario, check your equipment, arrange the documentation and radiographs, check that your patient is made up appropriately, and rehearse and brief your patient. **Faculty should allow at least 45 minutes for preparation before the sessions starts.**

Making the scenario as realistic as possible is vital to help the candidate feel that the process is real. It is difficult to write a scenario that covers all potential ages and shapes of patient models yet remains interesting, so the instructor must be ready to change any inappropriate points, eg the patient's sex. There will be few, if any, of these and they will be minor, so do not let them become an issue. Orientate the participant to the charts as necessary with respect to current dates and times. Start by reassuring the participant – introduce the scenario as an opportunity for the candidate to demonstrate how they can integrate all their knowledge – and take enough time in your briefing to settle the participant down.

Start with part 1 of each scenario. They are designed to test a mixture of skills, including factual knowledge on a range of topics, practical skills learned and organisational and communication skills. All participants should write a plan of action at some point in the scenario. The emphasis is best placed on 'what would the participant do now?', rather than too much on underlying theory. However, there is no need to limit questioning or discussion strictly to course material. This part of the course should form a link with real practice and it is reasonable to ask questions that the candidate should be able to answer from their general reading. Sometimes participants get to know the scenario from colleagues who have attended the CCrISP course already. It is the way in which the participant assesses and manages the patient, rather than whether or not they reach a particular diagnosis, that is important – and it can be worth pointing this out.

Each candidate should be taken through the material to complete the first two parts of the case scenario. With practice, the instructor will learn to control the pace of the scenarios and to adjust the pressure on the participant to enable this. The slow participant can be encouraged (eg by offering a further deterioration in condition) and the runaway slowed down (eg by asking for further detail with appropriate questions) in the time allowed. A few common pitfalls have emerged:

- Participants who are unwilling to role play may need encouragement to actually do things (such as listen to the chest or examine the abdomen). Avoid the situation of 'a viva over the patient' at all costs as this not a simulated moulage test.

- Some participants become stuck at the immediate assessment stage, performing a seemingly never-ending 'ABCDE assessment' as vital signs have not completely normalised. This is not realistic and they should be encouraged to progress to full patient assessment once adequate initial resuscitative measures are under way.

- Observing a stronger colleague is an important way for weaker participants to learn, so on the first and third runs (when you have a choice of candidates), pick the stronger one to perform first. This should be discussed with the course director in advance.

It is important that time is kept aside (within the 45 minutes) for feedback about performance, as this is one of few opportunities that doctors in training get to receive feedback about their clinical performance from otherwise independent seniors. Limit the scenario to about 35–40 minutes and let the other participant introduce a few positive aspects about the performance they have witnessed. Be ready to control the feedback so that the right balance between things done well and areas for improvement is achieved. The feedback can be as important as the performance – without it, the episode will be less meaningful for the participant.

The assessment sheet that links to the case should be used to assess performance – this is important for the feedback participants need at the end of their assessment or at the end of the course. Together with their performance in practical sessions, this will form their evaluation. Particular care needs to be taken in documenting reasons why candidates have performed poorly and each element of the assessment should be completed. Do not miss out elements of assessment in each part, eg the communication episode, as the assessment is criterion specific and to be certain that candidates who pass the course have reached the same standard it is necessary to ensure that all candidates have received a similar degree and scope of testing.

Timeline

Scenario	35–40 minutes
Feedback	5–10 minutes

Resources

▶ Faculty handbook and supporting notes;

▶ CCrISP system of assessment;

▶ equipment list as for simulated patient scenarios.

Do not leave this manual lying around for students to see.

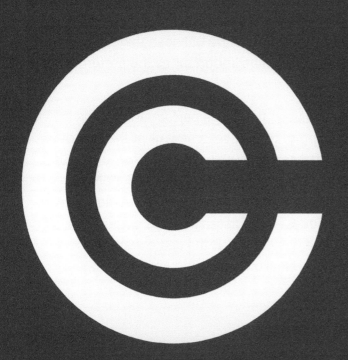

Practical session
Moulage scenario 1

Introduction

This scenario is in three parts and describes a postoperative vascular patient who has undergone an elective infrarenal aortic aneurysm repair with a tube graft.

Duration	45 minutes
Style	Practical
Faculty	Two
AV	NA

Objectives

- To carry out a systematic assessment.

- To understand the value of sequential assessment and reassessment.

- To understand the management of dysrhythmias.

- To understand the importance of identifying and treating the underlying cause of dysrhythmia.

- To be aware of severe wound infections/MRSA.

Timeline

Scenario	35 minutes
Feedback	10 minutes

Resources

▶ Faculty handbook and supporting charts and notes:

▶ CCrISP system of assessment poster;

▶ equipment list as for simulated patient scenarios.

Background information

- The patient is a 72-year-old man.

- Three days after elective AAA repair (tube graft) and back on surgical ward.

- First day spent on ITU – no problems.

- Second day spent on HDU – no problems.

- Medical history includes ischaemic heart disease, hypertension, mild angina, mild renal impairment (creatinine 140), ex-smoker and a duodenal ulcer years ago.

- Drugs include bendrofluazide 2.5 mg daily, atenolol 100 mg daily and GTN spray.

At the start of the scenario, he is 3 days post operation and doing well on the surgical ward. He is on free fluids and due to start a light diet. He has an IVI, urinary catheter and epidural. He then becomes acutely unwell.

The following significant postoperative events occur:

Part 1: He develops **atrial fibrillation** with mild hypotension 3 days postoperatively on the surgical ward. The participant is asked to resuscitate and manage the patient.

Part 2: He is transferred to the HDU and his arrhythmia is treated with amiodarone, a potassium infusion and recommencement of his beta blocker. The participant is asked to review the patient on the HDU. He is much improved but his urine output is poor and his creatinine has risen. The candidate should be asked about suitability for discharge back to the surgical ward.

Part 3: On postoperative day 6 he develops a wound infection, swinging pyrexia and progressive renal failure in part caused by NSAIDs. The participant is asked to reassess the patient and manage him.

Documents available

1. Atrial fibrillation with hypotension on the ward 3 days post operation (Saturday)

▶ 2.6.0 History sheet 1.

▶ 2.6.1 History sheet 2.

▶ 2.6.2 Prescription chart 1.

▶ 2.6.3 Patient observation chart 1.

▶ 2.6.4 Anaesthetic notes.

▶ 2.6.5 Chest X-ray.

▶ 2.6.6 Echocardiogram (preoperative).

▶ 2.6.7 Echocardiogram (now).

▶ 2.6.8 Blood results 1.

2. Review next morning (Sunday)

▶ 2.6.9 Patient observation chart 2 (from HDU).

▶ 2.6.10 Blood results 2.

3. Subsequent wound infection and renal compromise (Tuesday)

▶ 2.6.11 Patient observation chart 3.

▶ 2.6.12 Prescription chart 2.

▶ 2.6.13 Blood results 3.

At least two communication episodes should be included.

Parts may be omitted or the depth of coverage varied as appropriate.

Please read the general instructions with regard to running the scenarios (including safety, teaching approach, rehearsal and assessment) in your faculty handbook.

Part 1: atrial fibrillation with hypotension on the ward 3 days post operation (Saturday)

Make-up directions for patient

- Sweaty and poorly perfused.
- Midline abdominal dressing.
- One IVI running, urinary catheter in place and on O_2 via nasal specs (2 L/min).
- Epidural in place and running – fentanyl and bupivacaine.

Brief for patient

- You are 3 days after a major operation on the main blood vessel in the abdomen.
- You are breathless and easily rousable but you feel faint.

Brief for participant

You are the surgical registrar on call and it is 6pm on the surgical ward of a teaching hospital. You have been asked to see Mr Wilson, who is 3 days following an elective AAA repair, and was doing well. He has just collapsed and is acutely unwell. His initial observations are a tachycardia of 130 bpm and a BP of 110/70 mmHg. The FY1 has sent some arterial blood gases on air.

Immediate assessment and management

On arrival the patient is sweating and shut down. He is able to talk and feels faint. The participant should use the CCrISP system of assessment as follows:

A Patent and protected: administer oxygen at 15 L/min. Monitor SaO_2 – unreliable signal.

B Increased respiratory rate (28/min). Chest movements OK. Trachea central. Percussion OK. Few bilateral crepitations in the lower zones.

C Pulse 130/min irregular. BP 110/70 mmHg. Looks pale. Peripheral shutdown – sweaty and poorly perfused. Capillary refill time 4 seconds. Drip not working well – needs replacing. Urine clear (not sure about urine output until chart review). Give fluid challenge (start at 10 mL/kg). The participant should draw blood for FBC, glucose, urea and electrolytes and cross-match. Arterial blood gases should also be taken.

D AVPU: alert, pupils OK, BM Stix 6, moves arms and legs.

E Undressed and lying down in bed.

At some stage the participant should examine the abdomen, either during assessment of circulation or at the end. The abdomen is soft and non-tender but somewhat distended. The wound should be inspected for infection (looks OK). A few bowel sounds are present. The nasogastric tube is out. The patient has an epidural, which should be identified and stopped, and the candidate should indicate that this probably accounts for the non-tender abdomen.

Full patient assessment

Chart review

The following charts are available if asked for:

▶ 2.6.0 History sheet 1.

▶ 2.6.1 History sheet 2.

▶ 2.6.2 Prescription chart 1.

   • Includes IV drip chart on back (8-hourly bags but no potassium supplements). Drip behind time. Atenolol and diuretic not given.

▶ 2.6.3 Patient observation chart 1.

   • Sudden increase in heart rate and small fall in BP. Increased respiratory rate.

   • Temperature OK. Urine output tailed off in last 2 hours.

▶ 2.6.4 Anaesthetic notes.

   • Preoperative creatinine 140. Significant vascular risk factors.

History and systematic examination

□ Age 72.

□ Medical history includes ischaemic heart disease, hypertension, mild angina, mild renal impairment (creatinine 140), ex-smoker and a duodenal ulcer years ago.

□ Drugs include bendrofluazide 2.5 mg daily, atenolol 100 mg daily and GTN spray.

□ Now 3 days after elective AAA repair (tube graft).

□ First day spent on ITU – no problems.

□ Second day spent on HDU – no problems.

□ Now back on surgical ward.

□ Examination of abdomen (if not already done).

□ Examine lower limbs – viable, no DVT.

Review results

The participant should indicate that the following investigations are appropriate:

2.6.8 Urgent blood results

HB	101 g/L
WCC	10×10^9/L
Platelets	246×10^9/L
Na$^+$	130 mmol/L
K$^+$	2.6 mmol/L
Urea	13 mmol/L
Creatinine	170 µmol/L (was 140 µmol/L)

Arterial blood gases (sent by FY1)

pH	7.30
PaO_2	8.1 kPa
$PaCO_2$	3.8 kPa
HCO_3^-	18 mmol/L
FiO_2	nasal specs
Base excess	−4 mmol/L
Lactate	1.9 mmol/L

2.6.5 Chest X-ray

Slight basal atelectasis. No gas under diaphragm despite recent laparotomy.

2.6.6 and 2.6.7 Echocardiograms

▪ Preoperative: shows sinus rhythm and beta-blocked.

▪ Now: fast AF.

Decisions and planning

The candidate should reassess the patient and find some improvement from the oxygen and fluids (saturation 93%, BP 130/70, better perfusion). If the candidate administers large amounts of colloid, the patient should become increasingly breathless. At some stage the candidate should realise that the patient is not hypovolaemic (and turn the fluids down) and should have identified ischaemic heart disease on the chart review. The significance of low potassium and the need to estimate serum magnesium should be noted. Discuss how K and Mg will be administered.

The participant should indicate that the patient remains unstable and that:

- anaesthetic/ICU help should be sought;

- the patient needs to be transferred to the HDU/ICU;

- the surgical consultant should be informed;

- it may be necessary to administer frusemide (the appropriateness of this should be discussed).

The candidate should diagnose dysrhythmia and appreciate the need for referral (it is not essential that the candidate knows the precise treatment of the dysrhythmia under these circumstances). However, better candidates may be aware of the algorithm for the treatment of atrial fibrillation and be able to discuss the relative merits of DC cardioversion and medical treatment.

In this case the patient was transferred to the HDU and treated with amiodarone.

Diagnosis required: special investigations

The cause is atrial fibrillation (atenolol not given and low potassium and magnesium) with hypotension that responds to fluids. A myocardial infarction should be excluded (serial ECG and cardiac enzymes).

The candidate should be asked about the treatment of atrial fibrillation and possible causes in a postoperative patient (most candidates know about thyrotoxicosis and rheumatic fever but do not appreciate commoner postoperative causes such as myocardial ischaemia/infarction, hypoxia, hypokalaemia and hypotension from any cause (bleeding, sepsis, peritonitis). Other causes should be excluded by ECG, erect chest X-ray, troponin, septic screen (blood cultures) and possibly ultrasound/CT of the abdomen.

Plan of action

- Discuss with ICU/HDU/anaesthetic team and institute treatment as advised.

- Check bloods and blood gases if not done.

- Check troponin and ECG serially.

- Septic screen.

- Order chest X-ray if not done.

- Check calcium and magnesium levels.

- Consider central venous pressure (CVP) line insertion – should not be performed unsupervised and the patient should be in a monitored environment.

- Plan to restart the epidural appropriately.

- Some candidates may still wish to perform abdominal ultrasound/CT to exclude bleeding and the risks and benefits of this should be discussed.

- If there is time, a good participant should be asked to discuss the role of the surgeon in treating cardiac problems on an anaesthetic-led HDU.

Communication skills

The candidate should be asked to telephone the ICU (where the ICU consultant is available and reviewing a patient) and ask for help. The ICU consultant may wish to suggest an initial cardiological review. A good candidate should suggest that this is not appropriate and that the patient is unstable and requires urgent ICU review.

Part 2: reassessment on HDU

It is now the next day. Emphasise that the patient is doing well. The candidate should be told that the patient has been treated on the HDU with the help of the ICU staff with potassium and magnesium correction and an amiodarone infusion. Digoxin was not used. He is in sinus rhythm again with a normal pulse and blood pressure. The plan is to stop the amiodarone and potassium infusions and commence oral potassium supplements and oral metoprolol. Troponin was normal.

He has an IVI, urinary catheter, CVP line and epidural. However, his urine output is poor and his creatinine has risen. The candidate should recognise that the patient, though stable, is at risk of developing further problems, particularly renal failure.

Make-up directions

- IVI.
- Urinary catheter.
- Epidural.
- CVP line.

Brief for patient

- You are conscious and able to talk.
- You feel 'much better'.

Brief for participant

The next morning, Sunday (day 4 after the operation), you are reviewing the patient on your round on the HDU. He has been treated on the HDU with the help of the ICU staff with potassium and magnesium correction and an amiodarone infusion. Digoxin was not used. He is in sinus rhythm again with a normal pulse and blood pressure. The plan is to stop the amiodarone and potassium infusions and commence oral potassium supplements and oral metoprolol. Troponin was normal. He has an IVI, urinary catheter. CVP line and epidural. You are asked to determine whether the patient is fit for discharge to the ward as there are other emergency cases planned for today which may need a bed on the HDU.

Immediate assessment and management

The candidate should reassess the ABCs:

A Patient talking, SaO_2 96% on 30% O_2.

B Trachea central, chest clear.

C Warm and well perfused. HR 86, sinus rhythm. BP 125/85. IVI in place.

D Alert, pupils normal.

E Undressed.

Full patient assessment

Chart review

2.6.9 The candidate should review the HDU chart.

Urine output is not ideal.

Examine fully

Abdomen fine, normal bowel sounds and flatus passed.

Legs/feet NAD.

Review results

2.6.10 Today's results are back

Hb	99 g/L
WCC	9.8×10^9/L
Platelets	231×10^9/L
Na^+	135 mmol/L
K^+	4.5 mmol/L
Urea	15 mmol/L
Creatinine	205 µmol/L
Ca^{2+}	2.10 mmol/L
Mg^{2+}	1.34 mmol/L

Arterial blood gases

pH	7.33
PaO_2	14.5 kPa
$PaCO_2$	4.5 kPa
HCO_3^-	21 mmol/L

FiO_2	2 L/min via nasal specs
Base excess	–4 mmol/L
Lactate	0.9 mmol/L
Troponin T	normal
CXR	OK. No failure.
ECG	Sinus rhythm.

(The chest X-ray and ECG are not available.)

Decisions and planning

The participant should conclude that the patient is stable. The only potential problems are the increase in creatinine and poor urine output. The plan should be to observe cardiac rate (off amiodarone) and urine output on the HDU for 24 hours and the participant should discuss this and the hazards and/or safety of early discharge back to the ward. Candidates should be asked to write a daily management plan. They may wish to seek a renal opinion at this stage and indicate avoidance of nephrotoxic drugs.

Daily management plan

At this stage ask the candidate to write an entry in the case notes in the form of a daily management plan. This should include the following:

- Mobilisation

- Physiotherapy

- Change LMWH to b.d. sodium heparin SC

  - check bloods and arterial gases

- Wound care

  - nutrition plan

  - continue potassium

  - watch urine output

  - review.

Communication skills

The surgical consultant in charge of the case telephones the HDU about the patient. The candidate should be asked to talk to the consultant on the phone and update him or her about the current situation and management plan.

Part 3: wound infection, swinging pyrexia, MRSA-positive swabs and renal impairment

The patient was discharged early from the HDU because of a bed crisis. It is now 2 days later and the patient is on the surgical ward. He has been doing well and all lines and the catheter and epidural have been removed. He is on a light diet and build-up drinks. He has had diclofenac for pain. However, he has now developed a severe wound infection. For the last 24 hours he has been feeling unwell with a fever, has had a rigor and is now acutely unwell. Renal failure is developing. The candidate is asked to review the patient.

Make-up directions

- Sweaty, poorly perfused.
- Wound infection (large pad dressing).

Brief for patient

- You have now developed a potentially serious wound infection.
- Shiver intermittently. Some shortness of breath. Your wound is tender.

Brief for candidate

The patient was discharged early from the HDU because of a bed crisis. It's now 2 days later. He has been doing well and all lines, catheter and epidural have been removed. He is on a light diet and build-up drinks. He has had diclofenac for pain. You are called to see the patient because he is pyrexial.

Immediate assessment and management

- Patent and protected, talking. SaO_2 93%. Give oxygen.
- Mildly dyspnoeic, respiratory rate 22/min. Trachea central. Chest clear.
- Poor perfusion, HR 110/min, BP 105/50. Needs IV access and administration of some crystalloid (10 mL/kg).
- OK.
- Further undressing not needed; cover up again.

Full patient assessment

Chart review

- 2.6.11 The patient observation chart shows pyrexia (39°C) and a drop in BP.
- Urine output has not been measured.

2.6.12 The prescription chart shows Voltarol for pain relief given once (PRN chart) – now stopped.

Examine fully

Reasonably well yesterday. Not so good today. Rigor started 45 minutes ago.

Abdomen: severe wound infection with leakage of pus and serous fluid. Surrounding cellulitis and partial wound breakdown. No peritonitis.

Review results

No new results from this morning yet.

The candidate should send samples of blood for baseline FBC, U&E.

Other routine cultures such as wound swabs should also be sent.

Reassessment

Responds well to O_2 and fluid challenge (had 1000 mL).

BP increased to 120/75, HR 95/min.

2.6.13 Blood results are now available.

Hb	9.1 g/L
WCC	19×10^9/L
Platelets	255×10^9/L
Na$^+$	149 mmol/L
K$^+$	6.7 mmol/L
Urea	30 mmol/L
Creatinine	512 µmol/L
Bicarbonate	13 mmol/L
Creatine phosphate	298 mg/L

Note: early warning score has not been filled in and this would have raised an alert of a developing problem.

Decisions and planning

The participant should determine whether the patient is stable or not. **He is not.**

Diagnosis required: special investigations

The patient has a significant degree of sepsis and the question is whether or not the severe wound infection is an adequate cause.

- Previous culture results should be chased. Swabs from the abdominal wound are MRSA positive.

- Look for other sources (chest, abdomen, peri-graft) depending on response and suspicion (CXR? CT?).

- However, inspection of the wound shows there to be extensive slough and necrosis – an adequate **immediate** cause.

The deterioration in renal function needs assessing and treating promptly:

- Renal referral.

- Check ABGs.

- Urgent correction of K (CaCl administration, insulin/dextrose infusion) and recheck levels.

- Urgent discussion with ICU about haemofiltration.

- Antibiotics with dose modification and discussion with microbiology, particularly with regard to the MRSA and underlying prosthetic graft.

- Surgical debridement of the wound – requires consultation with seniors.

Communication skills

The patient's wife asks to discuss the current problems and expresses particular concern having heard that the swabs are MRSA positive. She wants to know what the implications are for her husband and why the infection has occurred.

This will demonstrate the following skills:

- explanation (factual communication)

- empathy (emotional management).

RCS

Moulage 1 assessment sheet

Candidate name		Assessors	

Assessment of knowledge
Candidates should provide commentary as they undertake the assessment to demonstrate knowledge and understanding of the theoretical basis and the implications of the knowledge for clinical practice.

Part 1	Score	Comments
Appropriate initial patient assessment.		
Appropriate full patient assessment: Request appropriate investigations.		
Appropriate full patient assessment: Interpret blood results, radiology and cardiac investigations.		
Assessment and plan of action; unstable patient, some improvement but transfer to HDU, exclude MI.		
Correct management of atrial fibrillation: electrolyte correction, digoxin/amiodarone, beta blocker and possible causes recognised: electrolytes, ischaemia, sepsis, (cardioversion).		
Other discussion of CVP line, (epidural management).		
Part 2		
Systematic initial patient assessment.		
Correct decision not suitable for discharge from HDU due to rising creatinine and falling urine output.		
Management plan includes fluid challenge, monitoring, possible renal opinion, avoid nephrotoxic drugs.		
Part 3		
Recognition of severity of sepsis and whether wound infection could be the cause: micro review, other sources, antibiotics.		
Recognition of deterioration in renal function: renal referral, ABGs, correct K, possible renal support.		
Discuss role of surgical debridement.		

Assessment of skills   Candidates should demonstrate effective practice in:

Part 1	Score	Comments
Appropriate immediate management of hypotension with ABCDE: oxygen & fluid challenge.		
Appropriate full patient assessment incl. chart reviews.		
Discussion of CVP lines: pros and cons (if appropriate).		
Telephone ICU consultant to make referral.		
Part 2		
Correct application of assessment system to patient on HDU in part 2.		
Formulation of HDU management plan for further surgical care includes physiotherapy, blood tests, nutrition, wounds and review.		
Discussion with surgical consultant.		
Part 3		
Explanation to relative: correct factual discussion and empathic manner.		

Scoring criteria   Assessment should consider actions performed as well as omitted.

Score	Criteria
A	Acceptable performance/knowledge in that area.
B	Minor Fault in performance or knowledge unlikely to materially affect patient outcome.
C	Potentially serious issue in knowledge or performance that may to lead to substantial and lasting impairment of patient function or increasing risk of dangerous outcome for patient or distress in relatives. Considerable prompting required to get any form of answer/action.
D	Serious/dangerous fault either by action or omission that might lead to death, serious damage or risk to patient of such damage or severe distress in relatives.

Overall score   Candidates must complete Parts 1 and 2 to pass the moulage, regardless of score.

Pass	More **A** than **B/C**.
Borderline	Equal balance of **A** and **B/C** (to be discussed at Faculty meeting).
Fail	One **D** in either part 1 or part 2; or mainly **C** in both parts.

Assessment sheets cannot be given to candidates, but can be used to give feedback on performance.

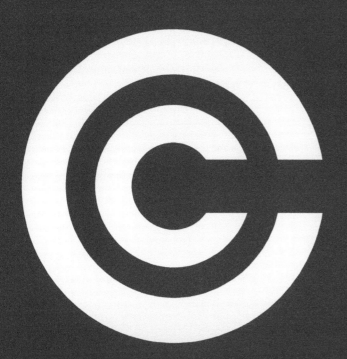

Practical session
Moulage scenario 2

Introduction

This scenario is in three parts and describes a postoperative general surgery patient who has undergone an emergency Hartmann's procedure. In the first part he has inadequate pain control and atelectasis. In the second part he develops sepsis associated with an intra-abdominal collection and chest infection. It is unlikely that candidates will get further than this but, if time permits, they can discuss sepsis care bundles and nutrition as part 3 of the scenario.

Duration	45 minutes
Style	Practical
Faculty	Eight
AV	NA

Objectives

- To carry out a systematic assessment.

- To understand the value of sequential assessment and reassessment.

- To understand atelectasis and prevention of postoperative respiratory complications.

- To understand the importance of identifying and treating the underlying cause of sepsis.

- To understand the value of a multidisciplinary team approach, including pain team, nutrition team and physiotherapy.

Timeline

Scenario	35 minutes
Feedback	10 minutes

Equipment

▶ Faculty handbook and pack containing charts and notes.

▶ CCriSP system of assessment poster.

▶ Equipment list as for simulated patient scenarios.

Background information

- It is the morning after the patient underwent a laparotomy for peritonitis due to perforated diverticular disease; an emergency Hartmann's procedure was performed.

- He was admitted at 7pm the previous evening with sudden onset of severe abdominal pain and a background of constipation.

- The patient is now on a level 1 surgical facility.

- Age: 50.

- Medical history includes obesity and asthma, for which he uses Ventolin and becotide inhalers. He is a smoker of 30/day.

- The following significant postoperative events occur:

   Part 1: The patient develops postoperative atelectasis **associated with inadequate analgesia**. With a background of obesity, smoking and asthma, he is at risk of respiratory complications. The procedure was performed in the middle of the night and it is not uncommon for adequate analgesia to be overlooked in such situations. Morphine PCA was prescribed and set up in recovery but the patient has not been using it. The candidate is asked to review, assess and manage the patient as the on-call surgical trainee taking over the Saturday day shift. At handover, the outgoing night trainee reported that the patient was stable overnight.

   Part 2: The patient is transferred to the HDU, pain control is improved and after 48 hours he is transferred to the ward. It is now day 6 and the patient develops **intra-abdominal sepsis and a left-sided chest infection**. He has been on the ward for the past 3 days. Progress has been slow. He has had a persistent ileus, is not mobilising well and is not willing to sit out, even with assistance. The abdominal wound is leaking haemoserous fluid.

   The candidate is informed on the morning ward round that the nurse is concerned about the patient's lack of progress and thinks he 'looks a bit grey today'. After a full assessment the candidate is expected to decide that the patient is unstable and requires a higher level of care plus targeted investigations to detect the source of sepsis. There should then be a discussion about source control.

   Part 3: Few candidates will have time for part 3 but in exceptional cases, if time permits, there can be a discussion about nutrition and sepsis care bundles relevant to the scenario.

Documents available

Atelectasis associated with inadequate analgesia

▶ 2.7.0 History sheet 1.

▶ 2.7.1 Operation note.

▶ 2.7.2 Drug prescription chart 1.

▶ 2.7.3 Patient observation chart.

▶ 2.7.4 Chest X-ray 1.

▶ 2.7.5 Blood results 1.

Ward round day 6: sepsis

▶ 2.7.6 History sheet 2.

▶ 2.7.7 Pain assessment chart.

▶ 2.7.8 Fluid balance chart 1.

▶ 2.7.9 Fluid balance chart 2.

▶ 2.7.10 Drug prescription chart 2.

▶ 2.7.11 Microbiology results.

▶ 2.7.12 Blood results 2.

▶ 2.7.13 Chest X-ray 2.

At least two communication skills should be included.

Parts may be omitted or the depth of coverage varied as appropriate.

Please read the general instructions with regard to running the scenarios (including safety, teaching approach, rehearsal and assessment) in your faculty handbook.

Part 1: atelectasis associated with inadequate analgesia (Saturday morning)

Make-up directions

- Pale, wearing hospital gown.
- Midline abdominal dressing.
- Green Venflon with IVI connected (1 litre Hartmann's running) and PCA attached but syringe full.
- Urinary catheter in place – clear urine in bag.
- On oxygen via mask.
- Pelvic drain connected to drainage bag – 50 mL serous fluid in bag.
- Stoma bag – left iliac fossa.

Brief for patient

You had an emergency operation last night for a perforated bowel. You have a background of asthma and are a smoker. The operation involved formation of a stoma.

You have been in a lot of pain overnight and have not been given any painkillers since return from theatre. You feel breathless and are in a lot of discomfort, able only to take very shallow breaths because of the pain. It is too painful to cough and difficult to move. You have been lying flat in bed all night, unable to sleep.

Brief for participant

You are the surgical trainee, just starting your daytime Saturday shift. It is 8.30am and you are asked to see a 50-year-old man who underwent an emergency laparotomy during the night for purulent peritonitis secondary to perforated diverticular disease.

The nurse tells you the patient is short of breath and in a lot of pain. He is on a level 1 surgical facility. He was previously a heavy smoker and he has a BMI of 38. The outgoing night trainee told you about the patient but said he had not been called through the night.

Immediate assessment and management

On arrival the patient is pale, breathless and in a lot of pain. He is lying flat on the bed. The candidate should use the CCrISP system of assessment as follows:

A   Patent and protected – talking, complaining of pain. Check the oxygen is at 15 l/min. The candidate should attach a pulse oximeter.

B   Increased respiratory rate (28/min), shallow breaths. Chest movements minimal. Trachea central. Percussion OK. Reduced air entry both lung bases. Unable to sit up and cough.

C   Pulse 120/min regular and good volume. BP 140/90 mmHg. Looks pale but the capillary refill time is 2–3 seconds. Urine output 29 mL in the past 60 minutes.

    Give fluid challenge (start at 10 mL/kg) and draw blood for FBC. Electrolyte profile, clotting, glucose and troponin. Arterial blood gases should also be taken.

D   AVPU: alert but in pain. Pupils OK, BM stix 6. Morphine PCA connected (unused).

E   In hospital gown, and lying down in bed. The candidate should examine the patient's abdomen at this stage, but the patient is in too much discomfort for a thorough examination. Midline wound, stoma in left iliac fossa – pink. Pelvic drain. Dressings not bloody; some haemoserous fluid in stoma bag. Temperature 37.9°C.

The participant should at this stage, if not already requested:

- attach pulse oximeter (SaO_2 92%);

- consider fluid challenge;

- check ABGs;

- order chest X-ray;

- order blood tests (FBC, electrolyte profile, clotting, glucose, troponin);

- order ECG.

The candidate may already recognise that inadequate analgesia is a major factor here and it would be very reasonable to request a morphine bolus to be given at this stage, before moving on to the full patient assessment.

Full patient assessment

Chart review

The following charts are available if asked for (2.7.0–2.7.3):

- History sheet 1 (2.7.0) and operation note (2.7.1):

    - These outline the preoperative history including comorbidity (heavy smoker, obese, on inhalers), and the late night operation, which describes extensive purulent peritonitis. The procedure was made difficult by the patient's size.

- Drug prescription chart 1 (2.7.2) (with *N* prescription on the back):

    - The patient is written up for his inhalers and has been given preoperative DVT prophylaxis and perioperative antibiotics. Morphine PCA is prescribed and a single litre of Hartmann's fluid written up and commenced at 4am.

- Patient observation chart (2.7.3):

    - Tachycardia, tachypnoea, high pain score, worsening NEWS. The sats have dropped gradually despite the oxygen delivery rate being increased through the night.

History and systematic examination

The patient is a 50-year-old man with the history as described before and further thorough examination reveals no new findings.

Review available blood results (2.7.5):

Hb	105 g/L
WCC	18.1×10^9/L
pH	7.42
Platelets	175×10^9/L
APPT	29.7 s
PT	11.3 s
Fibrinogen	1.8 g/L
ABG on 5 L/min	
PaO_2	10.1 kPa
$PaCO_2$	5.6 kPa
HCO_3^-	25.2 mmol/L
BE	−1.7 mmol/L
Lactate	1.5 mmol/L
Na^+	142 mmol/L
K^+	4.6 mmol/L
Urea	5.8 mmol/L

Creatinine	89 µmol/L
Albumin	24 g/L
Amylase	Normal
Glucose	5.4 mmol/L
Troponin T	Normal
ECG	sinus tachycardia
Chest X-ray 1 (2.7.4)	slight bilateral basal atelectasis, nothing else.

Decisions and planning

By now the candidates should have realised the importance of analgesia. If they have not given any analgesia, the patient could continue to deteriorate. Either way, the candidate should now reassess the patient. If analgesia has been given, the patient may be slightly more comfortable and the sats may have picked up slightly.

Participants should start to consider a plan of action.

The candidate should indicate that the patient is unstable.

Diagnosis required – special investigations

Further imaging at this stage is probably unnecessary. Some participants may want to arrange a CT scan, but this will be unhelpful and potentially dangerous in an unstable patient. The key here is to get adequate analgesia and reassess the patient fully when the pain is controlled. The candidates should all be aware that there may be underlying problems contributing to the pain, but it is clear in this case that analgesia has been inadequate. They should consider a full infection screen as part of the plan of action below.

Plan of action

The candidate should indicate that the patient remains unstable, hypoxic and in pain:

- continue with high-flow oxygen;

- nebulisers;

- infection screen – blood, urine, sputum if possible;

- physiotherapist review;

- improve pain control (ask for help, give further patient bolus analgesia, increase PCA dose);

- consider higher level of care;

- inform surgical consultant.

Communication skills

The candidate should indicate a need to call the surgical consultant and the outreach service. Some hospitals may not have outreach at the weekend, so discussions with anaesthetists and/or critical care are acceptable alternatives. At least one communication episode should take place here, though there is the potential to assess two:

 Communication with the outreach service about the appropriateness of transfer to a level 2 facility.

 Communication with the surgical consultant, who does not consider this to be a surgical problem as it is too soon after surgery, and instead considers that the chest is most pressing issue. The participant should then consider involving the outreach service, an anaesthetist and a critical care specialist.

The patient is transferred to the HDU, pain control is improved and after 48 hours in the HDU he is transferred to the ward.

Part 2: sepsis

It is now day 6. The patient spent 48 hours on the HDU before being transferred back to the ward. He has been on the ward for the past 3 days. Progress has been slow, though he has been stable. He has had a persistent ileus, is not mobilising well and is not willing to sit out, even with assistance. The abdominal wound is leaking haemoserous fluid.

He becomes unwell with intra-abdominal sepsis, an intra-abdominal collection and left chest infection. It is your routine ward round and the charge nurse asks the candidate to see the patient: the nurse is concerned at the lack of progress and reports that the patient 'looks a bit grey today'.

Make-up directions

 Sweaty, poorly perfused.

 Pale.

 Drain has been removed.

 Urinary catheters and Venflon still in place, with IVI connected.

 Midline dressing/stoma bag still attached.

 No oxygen mask.

Brief for patient

 It is now day 6 and you have been progressing very slowly.

 You have not felt well since the procedure but feel much worse this morning, because you have developed an infection.

 You have quite a lot of pain in the left side of the abdomen and you feel sick, hot and a bit short of breath.

Brief for candidate

The patient has been on the ward since transferring from the HDU 3 days ago. Progress has been slow. He has had a persistent ileus and has not been mobilising well and is not willing to sit out, even with assistance. The abdominal wound has been leaking haemoserous fluid.

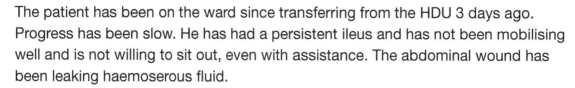

It is your routine ward round and the charge nurse has asked you to see the patient, having just changed the dressing. The nurse is concerned at the lack of progress and thinks the patient 'looks a bit grey today'.

Immediate assessment and management

A   Patent and protected, talking. Give high-flow oxygen and connect a sats probe (89% on air).

B   Mildly dyspnoeic, respiratory rate 20/min, trachea central. Chest: reduced air entry, left base and midzone. Dull to percussion, left base.

C   Poor perfusion, HR 130 /min, BP 85/40. Urine output 25 mL in the last hour. Needs IV access and administration of a crystalloid fluid challenge (10 mL/kg). Bloods should be taken at this stage.

D   Listless but responsive to voice, pupils normal.

E   Diffuse left-sided abdominal pain and tenderness, lower third of wound mildly inflamed, serous fluid, stoma looks OK, pelvic drain has been removed. Temperature 38.4°C.

The participant should at this stage, if not already requested:

- give high-flow oxygen;
- attach an oximeter;
- give a fluid challenge;
- order blood tests (FBC, U&E, clotting, group and save, troponin, amylase);
- order cultures – wound, urine and blood;
- send a blood sample for gas analysis;
- order a portable chest X-ray;
- order an ECG.

Full patient assessment

Chart review

The following charts are available if asked for (2.7.6–2.7.10):

- History sheet 2 (2.7.6)

- Pain assessment chart (2.7.7):

  Shows tachycardia, pyrexia, falling BP and sats. The NEWS has suddenly risen to 9.

  These confirm that the patient has been slow to progress. He had been vomiting during the previous day and the last entry is from the charge nurse, who has requested senior review.

- Drug prescription chart 2 (2.7.10) with IV drip chart on back:

  The drug chart shows that the antibiotics were stopped on day 3; he has been receiving thromboprophylaxis and inhalers. The fluid has generally been running behind schedule and he is currently prescribed 1 litre of crystalloid 12-hourly. Potassium supplements have not been prescribed.

- Fluid balance charts 1 and 2 (2.7.8 and 2.7.9):

  These show that the patient has been vomiting and taking small amounts of fluid orally supplemented by 80 mL/h IV. The urine output has been poor and is now less than 20 mL/h.

History and systematic examination

The candidate should fully examine the abdomen and check the wound and stoma at this point if he or she has not already done so earlier.

Review results

- Blood results 2 (2.7.12)

Hb	91 g/L	pH	7. 26 (FiO_2 0.8)
WCC	2.5×10^9/L	PaO_2	8.1 kPa
Platelets	103×10^9/L	$PaCO_2$	3.4 kPa
PT	14.3 s	HCO_3^-	15.2 mmol/L
APPT	35.3 s	BE	−9.7 mmol/L
Fibrinogen	1.2 g/L	Lactate	2.6 mmol/L
Na^+	137 mmol/L		
K^+	3.4 mmol/L		
Urea	11.3 mmol/L		
Creatinine	123 µmol/L		
Albumin	18 g/L		
Amylase	Normal		
Glucose	4.8 mmol/L		
Troponin T	Normal		

- Microbiology results (2.7.11)

Coliforms have been cultured from abdominal pus and blood; sputum contains mouth flora only.

  Chest X-ray 2 (2.7.13)

Opacity left base, probable consolidation (effusion?) at left base.

  ECG

Unchanged (not available).

Decisions and planning

The candidate should indicate that the patient is unstable and needs to be moved to a higher level of care (at least level 2).

The candidate should already have given oxygen and fluids and plan to give antibiotic cover and should consider calling the microbiology department for advice as the microbiological report suggests sensitivity to meripenem.

A full reassessment is required to establish how the patient is responding to the oxygen and fluid resuscitation.

The patient should respond partially to a fluid challenge in terms of blood pressure and urine output but remain unstable.

The surgical consultant should be informed about the patient's condition.

Diagnosis required – special investigations

The candidate should discuss the need for abdominal and thoracic imaging.

Options are ultrasound on the higher-level facility or CT. If CT is discussed, the stability of the patient and escort to scan should be considered. CT would be preferable and could be combined with CT-guided drainage of any intra-abdominal collection and/or infected pleural effusion.

Definitive treatment

Definitive treatment will involve CT-guided drainage of any collection, or laparotomy depending on the extent and anatomical site of any collections.

Summary: plan of action

Ask the candidate to summarise their plan for the patient, which should include:

  continued fluid resuscitation and oxygen;

  consideration of nebulisers and physiotherapy;

  analgesia;

  nutrition (this will need to be considered once the patient is on a higher level of care);

- antibiotics and repeat all cultures if not already performed;

- regular reassessment and observation;

- communication with:

  - higher level of care

  - consultant surgeon

  - radiology after discussion with consultant surgeon

  - microbiology

  - patient/relatives

- documentation of findings and plan in the case notes.

Communication skills

Use a further communication scenario if only one assessment was made in part 1 of the scenario. The patient asks that you tell his brother what is happening. The participant needs to communicate effectively and empathetically.

Part 3: optional discussion on care bundles and nutrition

If there is time, a strong participant can discuss the role of sepsis care bundles and total parenteral nutrition (TPN). This patient is going to require nutritional support once transferred to the higher level of care and the options/requirements should be discussed.

RCS

Moulage 2 assessment sheet

Candidate name		Assessors	

Assessment of knowledge   Candidates should provide commentary as they undertake the assessment to demonstrate knowledge and understanding of the theoretical basis and the implications of the knowledge for clinical practice

Part 1	Score	Comments
Appropriate initial patient assessment.		
Appropriate full patient assessment: Request appropriate investigations.		
Appropriate full patient assessment: Interpret blood results, radiology and cardiac investigations.		
Assessment and plan of action; recognise patient unstable, give analgesia, saline/bronchodilator nebs.		
Correct management of instability: recognise CT scan not appropriate, analgesia plan, infection screen, consider higher level care, physio review.		
Part 2		
Appropriate systematic patient assessment.		
Correct decision to move to higher level of care due to sepsis and inform seniors.		
Management plan includes micro review, antibiotic cover, imaging of abdomen and thorax or ultrasound scan.		
Part 3		
Discussion of sepsis care bundles and nutritional support.		

Assessment of skills Candidates should demonstrate effective practice in:

Part 1	Score	Comments
Appropriate immediate management within ABCDE: oxygen and fluid challenge.		
Appropriate full patient assessment.		
Discussion with outreach team for transfer to level 2 facility, or Telephone surgical consultant to inform and excludes surgical problem.		
Part 2		
Correct application of assessment system to patient, with appropriate blood tests, cultures, CXR and ECG.		
Discussion with brother: correct factual discussion in empathic manner or, discussion with consultant (radiology or ICU).		
Part 3		
Appropriate immediate management within ABCDE: oxygen and fluid challenge.		

Scoring criteria Assessment should consider actions performed as well as omitted.

Score	Criteria
A	Acceptable performance/knowledge in that area.
B	Minor Fault in performance or knowledge unlikely to materially affect patient outcome.
C	Potentially serious issue in knowledge or performance that may to lead to substantial and lasting impairment of patient function or increasing risk of dangerous outcome for patient or distress in relatives. Considerable prompting required to get any form of answer/action.
D	Serious/dangerous fault either by action or omission that might lead to death, serious damage or risk to patient of such damage or severe distress in relatives.

Overall Score

Candidates must complete Parts 1 and 2 to pass the moulage, regardless of score.

Pass	More **A** than **B/C**.
Borderline	Equal balance of **A** and **B/C** (to be discussed at Faculty meeting).
Fail	One **D** in either part 1 or part 2; or mainly **C** in both parts.

Assessment sheets cannot be given to candidates, but can be used to give feedback on performance.

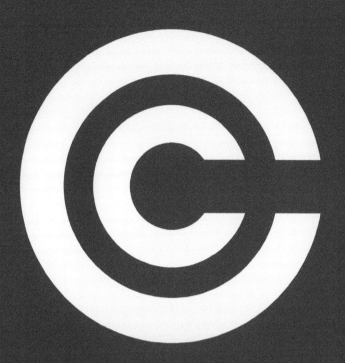

2.8

Practical session
Moulage scenario 3

Introduction

This scenario describes a patient with multiple medical problems and a large unruptured aneurysm. It is in three parts and most candidates will complete parts 1 and 2, with the 3rd part being available for the 'best' candidates, whose knowledge of enhanced recovery will be tested.

Learning outcomes

At the end of this session, the candidate will be able to:

- demonstrate how to carry out systematic assessment of a critically ill patient;

- understand the value of instituting early resuscitative measures with monitoring and reassessment with the establishment of a definitive management plan;

- manage a patient with a large uncomplicated aneurysm, hypotension and acute kidney injury;

- demonstrate in practice the principles of managing a patient with severe sepsis;

- discuss the components of planning pre-, intra- and postoperative care for this patient's large aneurysm with respect to the principles of enhanced recovery after surgery.

Timeline

Scenario   35 minutes

Feedback   10 minutes

Equipment

▶ Faculty handbook and supporting charts and notes.

▶ CCrISP system of assessment poster.

▶ equipment list as for simulated patient scenarios.

Documents available

▶ 2.8.0 Observation chart 1.

▶ 2.8.1 Fluid chart 1.

▶ 2.8.2 Prescription chart 1.

▶ 2.8.3 Admission note.

▶ 2.8.4 Chest X-ray 1.

▶ 2.8.5 ECG.

▶ 2.8.6 CT angiogram.

▶ 2.8.7 Blood results from DGH (district general hospital).

▶ 2.8.8 Observation chart 2.

▶ 2.8.9 Fluid chart 2.

▶ 2.8.10 Prescription chart 2.

▶ 2.8.11 FY1 notes.

▶ 2.8.12 FBC, U&E, cultures.

▶ 2.8.13 U/S renal tract.

▶ 2.8.14 CT scan.

▶ 2.8.15 Chest X-ray 2.

▶ 2.8.16 Serial bloods since admission.

Faculty notes

This scenario is in three stages.

In the first stage, a 75-year-old patient is transferred to the vascular unit from an outlying hospital for initial management of abdominal pain and acute kidney injury against a background of recent acute on chronic limb ischaemia that had been surgically treated. The history includes abdominal aortic aneurysm (AAA), renal stones, chronic pancreatitis, treated hypertension, three previous myocardial infarctions and a CVA 3 years ago). The patient is alert and talking and has a normal pulse, but is hypotensive and the blood creatinine level is markedly raised. An AAA is palpable but is non-tender. CT at the original hospital showed a 6.5 cm AAA with no sign of a leak, pancreatic calcification and renal stone disease. A combination of factors may be responsible for this presentation and treatment in accordance with CCrISP principles will improve the patient's condition. The diagnosis is essentially ureteric colic with an acute kidney injury exacerbated by the recent contrast study angiography. Providing on-going fluid resuscitation and oxygen are administered, antihypertensives/nephrotoxins are stopped and appropriate monitoring established, the patient will improve to the point of being almost ready for discharge.

The second stage is the day of planned discharge home when the patient suddenly deteriorates with signs of sepsis and shock. Ultrasound and repeat CT show the AAA to be intact, but a large right pyonephrosis is noted, as a result of which the patient should be referred to urology for urgent drainage of the pyonephrosis. Stenting and stone removal is carried out and the patient is prepared for discharge home.

The final stage requires a discussion with the patient (with or without relatives present) regarding the timing of elective AAA repair and could include discussion of preoperative planning, perioperative care and expected recovery and outcome (to include some of the principles of enhanced recovery after surgery).

Part 1

Brief for the actor

You are a 75-year-old patient admitted with left flank and abdominal pain and nausea. You have a history of heart attacks and stroke (but recovered well), kidney stones and chronic pancreatitis. You remain a heavy smoker. Two months ago you were in the same hospital (40 miles from home) with a painful leg that required an operation. You also have an aneurysm of your aorta and are waiting for this to be repaired. Your current pain feels like your kidney stones playing up, although you have had some diarrhoea and vomiting and you feel generally unwell.

Make-up instructions

The patient looks a bit sallow and pale. There is a healed scar in the right groin and thigh. There is also an open wound, 6 cm long and 1.5 cm wide, which is superficial and sloughy, on the medial aspect of the right knee, but with no sign of surrounding cellulitis.

Brief to the candidate

You are the surgical specialist registrar covering the admissions to the vascular unit and the night-time registrar hands over a 75-year-old patient, E Smyth, who was transferred from an outlying hospital A&E, having presented there with a history of abdominal and left flank pain and vomiting. There is a drip running and 2 litres of oxygen via nasal specs. The patient is alert with a pulse of 70, but is hypotensive. The charge nurse would like you to assess this patient first on your ward round.

Immediate management

A   Clear, with the patient alert.

B   Talking in full sentences, nasal cannulae in place attached to wall oxygen at 2 L/min. Trachea central and chest expansion equal. Normal percussion note and breath sounds. Saturations 96%. Candidate should increase oxygen to 15 L/min through a non-rebreathing mask.

C   Pulse 76 and regular, BP 80/50, capillary refill time 4 seconds, cool peripheries. A second IV access, blood tests including ABG, blood cultures and lactate should be obtained. Fluid challenge given (500 mL normal saline/Hartmann's).

D   Pupils normal and reacting equally, patient alert and orientated, blood sugar 4.5 mmol/L. Patient has a catheter in place, 17 mL urine in past hour.

E   Non-tender palpable aneurysm in the epigastrium. No guarding. The sloughy wound below the medial aspect of the right knee is noted, but there is no sign of cellulitis.

Management needs

The patient requires 15 l/min oxygen, IVI, blood tests, ECG, fluid replacement, and monitoring of oxygen sats, pulse and BP and urine output. The candidate should state that a chest X-ray is required as part of the full patient assessment and order one if not done previously.

Full patient assessment

2.8.0 Observation chart. The candidate should note the gradual drop in BP, probably associated with inadequate fluid resuscitation as the patient is apyrexial.

2.8.1 Fluid chart. The candidate should note that the drop in urine output is relatively recent.

2.8.2 Drug chart. The candidate should note the concerns of even PRN diclofenac and should recommend cancelling that prescription. In the regular meds section, the candidate should indicate that bisporolol and perindopril should be discontinued at present in view of the patient's BP and consider whether or not to continue aspirin.

2.8.3 Admission note. The candidate should note that patient has deteriorated since the FY1 clerking and that there has been suboptimal fluid resuscitation based on a spurious history of 'heart disease' and left basal crackles. The candidate should also note the lack of clear objective parameters to trigger further review.

2.8.4 Chest X-ray 1. The candidate should note that the chest X-ray is not normal: there is evidence of chronic chest disease.

2.8.5 ECG. This shows evidence of previous infarction.

2.8.6 CT angiogram from outlying hospital (two representative slices from the scan). There is no evidence of a leak. The candidate should note the contrast and the effect this may have had on subsequent renal function and evidence of an AKI.

2.8.7 Blood results from outlying hospital. The candidate should note the lack of evidence of infective markers and clear rise in creatinine consistent with an AKI.

Decisions and planning

Unstable.

Actions

Monitor vital observations and fluid input and output.

Check serum biochemistry parameters, FBC and CRP and monitor regularly.

Stop nephrotoxins.

Stop antihypertensives.

Prescribe analgesia for ureteric colic.

Medical management – ask for renal advice.

- Level of care? The candidate should note the risk of further deterioration and the potential need for renal support if action is not taken now to ensure adequate resuscitation.

- Communication episode: the candidate should phone the consultant, outlining the findings and the management plan.

Part 2

Brief for the actor

You have made good progress for the past 2 days, which includes passing a stone in your urine, leading to relief of your pain, and you are preparing to go home. You are suddenly unwell again and are shivering, with further abdominal and right flank pain, and you are mildly confused, thinking that you were already at home last night.

Make-up instructions

The patient looks flushed and sweating, but otherwise as before, with the right leg wound showing no sign of spreading cellulitis. No IV access or catheter is in place as the patient is about to be discharged.

Brief to the candidate

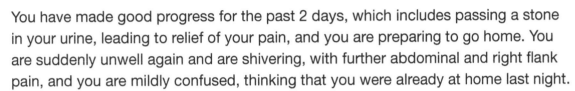

You attend the ward round 2 days later and are surprised when the charge nurse asks you to review the patient before the round begins. Your previous management plan has worked and, having passed a calculus in his urine the previous day and with improving renal function, you were expecting the patient to go home later today after a further check of renal function. However, the patient has suddenly become unwell, with further abdominal pain, fever and confusion.

Initial assessment

A   The airway is patent and the patient is talking, but slightly breathless.

B   RR 27/min, chest expansion equal, percussion note and breath sounds normal. The candidate should have given 15 L/min oxygen via a non-rebreathing bag at this point.

C   Pulse 100, BP 150/85, warm peripheries, capillary refill time 3 seconds. No IV access. The candidate should indicate that IV access is needed and a fluid challenge should be given.

D   The patient responds to voice, but is mildly confused, believing that last night was spent at home. PERLA. BM 5.6 mmol/L.

E   Temperature 38°C, abdomen soft with a palpable, but non-tender AAA, flank tenderness (R > L).

Management needs

The patient needs 15 L/min oxygen via a non-rebreathing mask, and oxygen sats should be monitored, as should temperature pulse, BP and RR. A fluid challenge should be given and bloods taken for tests including measurement of lactate.

Full patient assessment

- 2.8.8 Observation chart 2. A sudden rise in temperature and CVS deterioration is consistent with systemic sepsis.

- 2.8.9 Fluid chart 2. Note that this is the chart of the previous 24 hours. IV access has been discontinued and the patient is no longer catheterised.

- 2.8.10 Prescription chart 2. Note that perindopril has been stopped and bisporolol omitted from the chart.

- 2.8.11 FY1 notes. The candidate should note that the FY1 has not carried out any investigations, or instigated any treatment, including antibiotics.

Decisions and planning

The patient is unstable. Further investigations are needed and urgent treatment for possible sepsis. The source of any sepsis should be investigated.

- 2.8.12 FBC, U&E, cultures (blood, urine, sputum, leg wound; everything possible), ABG.

- 2.8.13 Ultrasound of renal tract.

- 2.8.14 CT scan.

- 2.8.15 Chest X-ray 2.

The candidate should indicate that they would administer broad-spectrum antibiotics at this point.

- If US asked for tell the candidate that it shows a dilated right renal pelvis,

- The chest X-ray does not indicate new pneumonia that would account for the patient's deterioration.

- 2.8.16 Serial bloods since admission. Serial bloods review shows that renal function has improved but is not yet back to previous normal. Candidates should consider whether US or CT would be less risky to kidneys and what they would do to further reduce risk of AKI with any repeat scan.

- Repeat CT scan shows an intact aneurysm, right hydroureter and hydro/pyonephrosis, with a calculus lodged in the distal right ureter and pancreatic calcification but no oedema or necrosis.

Communication episode

▫ The candidate could refer the patient to radiology to arrange percutaneous nephrostomy.

▫ Alternatively, the candidate could phone the urology team to ask them to take over the patient's care.

Management

▫ Following percutaneous right nephrostomy the patient should be transferred to the urology department for endoscopic ureterolithotomy and ureteric stent placement. Once the stent is removed you are asked to see the patient before discharge.

▫ If the candidate requests it, the nephrostogram showing a pigtail stent in the pelvis can be shown.

Part 3

▫ The patient and/or relatives want to see you before the patient goes home to find out what you plan to do about the patient's abdominal aortic aneurysm. The discussion will be with a member of faculty role-playing the family member regarding preparation for this major operation.

This is a complex topic, and the discussion should cover the timing of surgery. A delay to allow recovery from this acute episode will allow the leg wound to heal, but waiting runs the risk of AAA rupture. In contrast, early intervention means that physiological reserve is low and there is a risk of graft infection in the presence of an existing open wound. Furthermore, cardiac and antihypertensive drugs will need to be re-instituted and it will be important to ensure that the AKI is fully resolved and kidney function is restored to premorbid levels as far as possible. The patient will need to attend a pre-assessment clinic with specialist anaesthetic involvement to undergo robust cardiorespiratory risk assessment and optimisation. The patient should be given preoperative advice, both verbal and written, about taking exercise and stopping smoking. The patient should also be given information about drug modulation, the role of the multidisciplinary team, perioperative care, for example recovery in the HDU/ITU (the duration of which will depend on whether the open or endovascular repair is carried out), return to drinking and eating, pain management and how long it will take before normal activity can be resumed following discharge from hospital (ERAS [Enhanced Recovery After Surgery] principles).

RCS

Moulage 3 assessment sheet

Candidate name		Assessors	

Assessment of knowledge

Candidates should provide commentary as they undertake the assessment to demonstrate knowledge and understanding of the theoretical basis and the implications of the knowledge for clinical practice.

Part 1	Score	Comments
Appropriate initial patient assessment.		
Appropriate full patient assessment: Request appropriate investigations.		
Appropriate full patient assessment: Interpret blood results, radiology and ECG.		
Written assessment and plan of action; recognise patient unstable, stop PRN and diclofenac, and omit bisoprolol and perindopril.		
Correct management of instability and AKI.		
Part 2		
Appropriate systematic patient assessment.		
Appropriate review of results and comes to conclusion of sepsis with possible renal tract source.		
Management plan includes micro review, antibiotic cover, imaging of abdomen and thorax or ultrasound scan.		
Part 3		
Discussion of risks and timing of surgery, anaesthetic pre-op assessment review, post op care.		

Assessment of skills

Candidates should demonstrate effective practice in:

Part 1	Score	Comments
Appropriate immediate management of hypotension within ABCDE: O_2 and fluid challenge of appropriate volume and timescale.		
Appropriate full patient assessment including noting BP drop from inadequate fluid resuscitation.		
Candidate sets clear parameters for review and asks for advice from renal team.		
Telephone surgical consultant to inform and excludes surgical problem.		
Part 2		
Correct application of assessment system to patient, with appropriate blood tests, cultures, CXR and ECG.		
Discussion with radiology or phone call to urology team to ask them to take over care.		
Part 3		
Assimilation of information, organising that information and communicating that information to the recipient		

Scoring criteria   Assessment should consider actions performed as well as omitted.

Score	Criteria
A	Acceptable performance/knowledge in that area.
B	Minor Fault in performance or knowledge unlikely to materially affect patient outcome.
C	Potentially serious issue in knowledge or performance that may to lead to substantial and lasting impairment of patient function or increasing risk of dangerous outcome for patient or distress in relatives. Considerable prompting required to get any form of answer/action.
D	Serious/dangerous fault either by action or omission that might lead to death, serious damage or risk to patient of such damage or severe distress in relatives.

Overall Score

Candidates must complete Parts 1 and 2 to pass the moulage, regardless of score.

Pass	More **A** than **B/C**.
Borderline	Equal balance of **A** and **B/C** (to be discussed at Faculty meeting).
Fail	One **D** in either part 1 or part 2; or mainly **C** in both parts.

Assessment sheets cannot be given to candidates, but can be used to give feedback on performance.

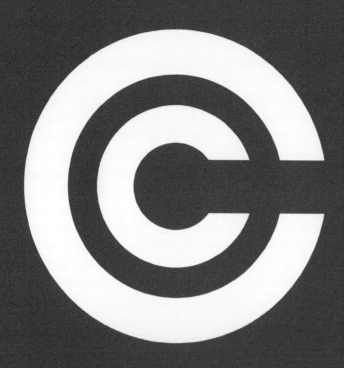

Group session
The virtual ward round

Background

The virtual ward round (VWR) runs in parallel with the practical management summative assessment, as the final session of the course. Half of the candidates take part in the VWR while the other half are being assessed. Unfortunately, this may detract from the importance of the VWR, particularly if participants are preoccupied with the forthcoming assessment or suffering a post-assessment lull. However, this arrangement is necessary to allow delivery of the course material within the allotted time and we must therefore focus on the content of the VWR to ensure that candidates remain motivated.

The VWR must accurately reflect situations that the candidates would expect to encounter at work. In an era of shift-based working patterns, accurate exchange of information between shifts is of paramount importance and we propose that the format of the VWR is modified to replicate a typical handover. This will allow the participants to focus on an increased number of patients with a greater range of clinical problems, drawing on all aspects of the CCrISP course. This combination of face validity and content validity will hopefully improve engagement with the VWR for all candidates.

Cases

We have provided 10 clinical cases from which the faculty can select eight for the VWR session. Each case consists of clinical notes on which the candidates must base their decisions. Not all cases are 'nightmare scenarios'; some are relatively straightforward to manage. We believe this case mix provides a greater validity for candidates.

Materials

▶ 2.9.0 Case 1: necrotising fasciitis in a patient with diabetes and a perianal abscess.

▶ 2.9.1 Case 2: ascending cholangitis (secondary to choledocholithiasis) causing confusion, which resulted in a fall and a fractured left neck of femur.

▶ 2.9.2 Case 3: symptomatic hypocalcaemia following a parathyroidectomy.

▶ 2.9.3 Case 4: high nasogastric output 1 week after laparotomy and adhesiolysis for small bowel obstruction; hypokalaemia and hypomagnesaemia.

▶ 2.9.4 Case 5: malignant otitis externa with skull base osteomyelitis and facial nerve involvement in an HIV-positive patient with diabetes.

▶ 2.9.5 Case 6: patient with cerebral palsy who underwent a laparotomy and adhesiolysis for small bowel obstruction 35 days previously; percutaneous endoscopic gastrostomy (PEG) aspirates are too high to allow enteral feeding but serial CT scans have shown no mechanical obstruction.

▶ 2.9.6 Case 7: elderly patient with COPD who has undergone repair of an incarcerated left inguinal hernia under local anaesthetic and has developed a respiratory acidosis (as a result of overoxygenation).

▶ 2.9.7 Case 8: patient with chronic pancreatitis and a history of schizophrenia, IV drug use and alcohol abuse who is abusive to members of staff and non-compliant with treatment.

▶ 2.9.8 Case 9: elderly patient with an obstructing ascending colonic tumour.

▶ 2.9.9 Case 10: brachial artery false aneurysm and compartment syndrome following coronary angiography.

Learning outcomes

At the end of this session, participants will be able to:

- demonstrate the ability to assimilate information about a variety of patients and use that information to formulate appropriate management plans;

- discuss these management plans with peers and prioritise patients according to their clinical needs;

- present these management plans to peers and faculty, and justify the decisions made.

Candidates

Eight (divided into two groups of four). The session will then be repeated for the remaining eight candidates.

Instructions

Each group will be presented with clinical information (notes, charts, radiology) about eight patients. Each candidate will take responsibility for two patients. See the following pages for a complete set of the documents given to participants.

Time available

75 minutes, allocated as follows:

- 5 minutes: introduction, division into two groups;

- 15 minutes: each candidate will review the clinical information (notes, charts, radiology) for two patients and formulate an appropriate management plan;

- 15 minutes: within each group of four, each candidate will give a brief summary of his or her patients together with the proposed plan and the group will then prioritise the plans for all eight patients;

- 10 minutes: each group will present their prioritised management plans to the other group/faculty (5 minutes for each group);

- 25 minutes: discussion (all);

- 5 minutes: debrief.

Case summaries

2.9.0 Case 1: necrotising fasciitis

The candidates should recognise that the presentation is not simply a perianal abscess that requires incision and drainage but a case of necrotising fasciitis that requires immediate resuscitation, antibiotics and urgent debridement in theatre. Advice may be sought from plastic surgeons and the microbiology team, and postoperatively the patient should be managed on an HDU. The patient should be counselled about the risks of extensive tissue loss (including amputation).

2.9.1 Case 2: ascending cholangitis and fractured neck of femur

This case concerns a patient with ascending cholangitis due to choledocholithiasis confirmed by magnetic resonance cholangiopancreatography (MRCP), which clearly demonstrates a distal common bile duct filling defect. This has resulted in sepsis and confusion, which has caused the patient to fall and sustain a fractured left neck of femur (displaced/intracapsular). The candidates must recognise that the patient needs on-going resuscitation, decompression of her biliary tree and hemiarthroplasty. However, there are risks associated with implanting metalwork in the presence of a bacteraemia and, therefore, biliary decompression via ERCP should be performed before orthopaedic surgery. This will require liaison with the general surgical and orthopaedic teams. Vitamin K should be given in line with local protocols. The patient's confusion will necessitate completion of a consent form 4, and the candidate should recognise that discussion with the patient's family/next of kin is good practice under these circumstances. The patient's falling urine output is a sign of severe sepsis and the candidates should identify the need for transfer to a higher level of care.

2.9.2 Case 3: hypocalcaemia

This case concerns a patient with symptomatic hypocalcaemia following a parathyroidectomy. The candidates should recognise the need for calcium replacement, which in this instance should be with intravenous 10% calcium gluconate (with ECG monitoring) until the patient is asymptomatic. Mild hypocalcaemia (> 1.9 mmol/L) can be treated with oral calcium supplements. Candidates may wish to discuss management with an endocrinologist or the on-call physician. The need for a calcium infusion to achieve normocalcaemia can be discussed. Calcium chloride can be used but it is more irritant to veins and should be administered via a central line.
The patient may require oral calcium treatment (eg 1-alfacalcidol) on discharge, with regular monitoring of adjusted serum calcium levels.

2.9.3 Case 4: persistent ileus, failure to progress

This case concerns a patient who is in 'status quo' – getting neither better nor worse. It is now day 7 after a laparotomy for adhesiolysis and the high nasogastric output should alert the candidates to the possibility of on-going intestinal obstruction. This may be secondary to electrolyte imbalances and the hypokalaemia and hypomagnesaemia should certainly be corrected via the IV route. Some candidates may wish to correct these abnormalities and monitor the patient over the next 24 hours to see if any improvement is observed. However, candidates should identify the need for imaging to exclude mechanical obstruction. The patient is haemodynamically stable and CT would be appropriate. The need for nutritional support must be recognised; total parenteral nutrition (TPN) via a dedicated central line should be discussed.

2.9.4 Case 5: malignant otitis externa

This is a case of malignant otitis externa with skull base osteomyelitis and facial nerve involvement (lower motor neurone lesion as evidenced by the loss of control of the frontalis muscle, leading to weak eye closure and diminished forehead wrinkling). Candidates should recognise that a history of diabetes mellitus and HIV infection are factors predisposing to malignant otitis externa and that the appearances at otoscopy (fleshy granulations in the external auditory meatus) are classical features. The fundamental principles of treatment involve glucose control, aural toilet and antibiotics (systemic and ototopic). Hyperbaric oxygen therapy may be useful in patients experiencing a poor response to treatment (or in cases of recurrence/complications). CT or MRI is useful in establishing the extent of soft-tissue inflammation and abscess formation. ENT surgeons and physicians specialising in HIV should be involved in the care of this patient at an early stage.

2.9.5 Case 6: cerebral palsy case conference

This is another case of a patient who is failing to progress. Postoperative CT has twice failed to demonstrate any mechanical obstruction but the small bowel remains dilated and PEG aspirates are high. The patient is currently receiving nutritional support via a Hickman line. If home TPN could be arranged then there would be no impediment to the parents taking their son home. However, it may be prudent to consider referral to a gastroenterologist/neurologist with an interest in cerebral palsy to explore any other management strategies for intestinal motility problems.

2.9.6 Case 7: respiratory failure with poor patient reserve

This case concerns a patient with COPD who has received too high a concentration of oxygen postoperatively, leading to a respiratory acidosis. Candidates should recognise that he needs non-invasive ventilatory support to treat his type 2 respiratory failure. This will require transfer to a higher level of care (either high dependency or a dedicated respiratory unit). However, given this patient's comorbidities and poor exercise tolerance, a discussion around DNACPR and appropriate ceiling of care should take place. There are other reasons for drowsiness and confusion postoperatively (electrolyte imbalances, alcohol withdrawal, opiates, hypoglycaemia, etc) and, although candidates may wish to exclude these, they should identify that this is primarily a respiratory problem.

2.9.7 Case 8: chronic pancreatitis

This patient has chronic pancreatitis as shown by the pancreatic calcification on CT. Her abusive behaviour is unacceptable and cannot be tolerated. If she wishes to remain in hospital to continue to receive analgesia then she must comply with the medical and nursing staff. However, candidates should recognise that the results of her investigations are reassuring, and plans could be made for discharge. She may require follow-up with the chronic pain and mental health teams and should be offered support for her alcohol and drug use.

2.9.8 Case 9: intestinal obstruction

This patient has an obstructing colonic tumour in the distal ascending colon. CT indicates that there is no local or metastatic spread, implying that a right hemicolectomy would be curative. However, candidates should recognise that there are significant risks associated with an emergency laparotomy in an 87-year-old patient. The situation should be discussed with the patient and, if he wishes to proceed with an operation, then an anaesthetic/intensive care review should be organised to assess his fitness for surgery. Candidates may discuss colonic stents but they are not currently recommended for right-sided colonic lesions.

2.9.9 Case 10: brachial artery aneurysm

This is a case of a brachial artery pseudoaneurysm due to an iatrogenic arterial puncture (from a coronary angiogram) complicated by the development of a forearm compartment syndrome with median nerve symptoms. In the absence of a compartment syndrome then ultrasound-guided compression with or without thrombin injection would be a reasonable strategy, but in this case the patient needs an emergency operation to (a) repair the false aneurysm and (b) relieve the pressure in the forearm via fasciotomies. Candidates should recognise the urgency of the situation and the need to involve vascular surgeons and cardiologists (to determine the type of stents inserted and the requirements for on-going antiplatelet treatment).

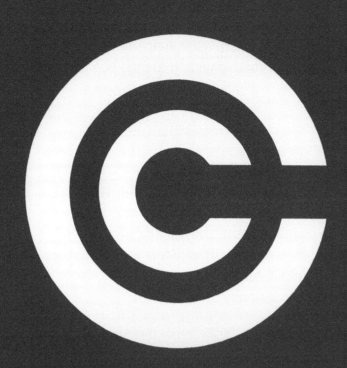

2.9.0

Case 1

6 September 08:30

Peter Smith: Surgical CT O/C
50 yr old ♂ with 4/7 history of painful perianal swelling
Last 24 h c/o ↑ing pain spreading across buttocks into L leg
Now feels unwell & feverish
No concerning lower GI symptoms or change in bowel habit

PMHx	SHx
HTN – amlodipine	Smoker – 20 cpd
IDDM – insulin glargine	Occasional EtOH
Ø MI, Ø CVA	Plasterer

Open R inguinal hernia repair (2000)

O/E
Temp 38.5°C
Pulse 110 BP 95/55
RR 16 BM 21
Abdo soft non-tender, obese (BMI 31)
Tender, tense, dusky perianal swelling @ 5 o'clock
Erythema across perineum, buttocks & L leg
2 blisters on L thigh

Impression
Perianal abscess with cellulitis

Plan
Needs I&D
Analgesia
NBM & IVI
D/w ST re theatre

P Smith
Peter Smith Bleep 430

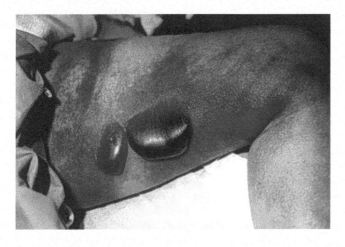

Charles Goldberg MD/UCSD

What would you do next?

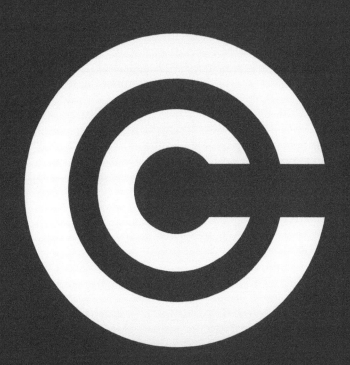

2.9.1

Case 2

4 September 8:15

<u>Nadia Khan: Surgical CT O/C</u>
74 yr old ♀ c upper abdominal pain & jaundice
2/7 h/o pain in RUQ c radiation →back
Assd nausea but no vomiting
Daughter told pt she 'looked yellow' yesterday
Dark urine and pale stools for ~1/52
Itching +++
No wt loss, no dysphagia, mild indigestion
Feels shivery

<u>PMHx</u>
PMR – prednisolone 5 mg od
TIA (2006) – aspirin 75 mg od, simvastatin 40 mg od
OA knees – paracetamol 1 g qds
NKDA

<u>SHx</u>
Never smoked
Alcohol rarely
Lives in bungalow; does own shopping, cleaning, etc.

<u>O/E</u>
Temp 38.5°C Pulse 105
BP 132/68
RR 24
HS 1+2
Few crackles at R base otherwise chest clear
Icteric

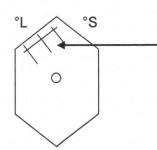

RUQ tenderness but no mass

No organomegaly / hernia

Courvoisier's sign −ve

DRE: pale stool on glove

<u>Impression</u>
Obstructive jaundice?GS/rule out pancreatitis

<u>Plan</u>
Admit to SAU
IV access and bloods
IVI
U/S abdomen

NK
Nadia Khan (CT Surgery)

4th September 11:00

Bloods

WCC 18.5 (neut 14.6)	Na 132	Alk Phos 822	CRP 320
Hb 112	K 3.6	ALT 324	Amylase 72
Plt 143	Creat 127	Bili 177	
Coag N	Urea 11	Alb 30	

Start antibiotics – 1.2g co-amoxiclav TDS

NK
Nadia Khan (CT Surgery)

4 September 15:00

Ultrasound report:
Thin walled gallbladder containing multiple small calculi. The liver is grossly normal. CBD is dilated at 11mm but no filling defect is identified. There is marked intrahepatic bile duct dilatation. The visualised pancreas is grossly normal but there is overlying bowel gas.

M. Thompson
M. Thompson (Sonographer)

4 September 16:40

Consultant review: Miss Edwards
For MRCP mane
Repeat bloods mane

James Bates
James Bates (FY1 Surgery)

5 September 08:00

WR Miss Edwards
Persistent RUQ tenderness
Seems confused this am
Temp 37.8
Pulse 110, BP 120/60
Plan: chase MRCP & continue with antibiotics
Can have clear fluids PO

James Bates
James Bates (FY1 Surgery)

5 September 15:00

Bloods

WCC 17.5 (neut 13.6)	Na 130	Alk Phos 956	CRP > 380
Hb 105	K 3.4	ALT 385	
Plt 187	Creat 110	Bili 185	
Urea 10	Alb 28		

James Bates
James Bates (FY1 Surgery)

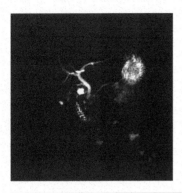

5 September 17:00

<u>WR ST6 Mr Chang</u>
Confused/V tender RUQ but not peritonitic
Temp 38.4 Pulse 105 BP 104/64
Blood cultures
Chase MRCP report
Catheterise
Input/output chart

James Bates
James Bates (FY1 Surgery)

6 September 05:00

<u>FY1 On Call: Sophie Barnes</u>
ATSP following fall when trying to get out of bed
Patient has been very confused; thinks she's in prison
Catheter wrapped round leg – urine output 70mL last 4 h
Found on floor by HCA
L leg now shortened and externally rotated
Needs urgent X-ray L hip

SASB
S. Barnes

6 September 07:30

X-ray reviewed:
L NOF

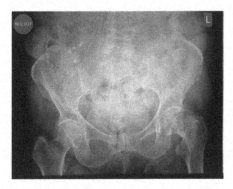

SASB
S. Barnes

What will you do now?

What will you ask others to do?

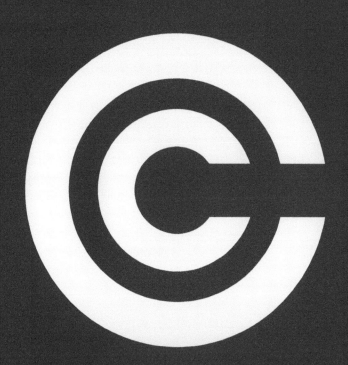

2.9.2

Case 3

4 September 18:00

FY1 Clerking
40 yr old ♀ admitted for elective parathyroidectomy
Several year history of constipation and abdominal pains treated with laxatives
Admitted to SAU earlier this year with R ureteric calculus (Rxed conservatively) and diagnosed
with hypercalcaemia (Ca 3.05) due to elevated PTH
U/S and sesta-MIBI scans revealed parathyroid hyperplasia
Hypercalcaemia treated with alendronate
No evidence of MEN

PMHx
Depression: fluoxetine
Allergic to penicillin (rash and swelling)

O/E
Pulse 90   Chest clear
BP 140/86   Abdomen soft but mildly tender in LIF
HS normal   No previous neck surgery

Bloods
Hb 120   Ca (adj) 2.7   Na 141
WCC 7.3   Alb 35   K 3.9
Plt 145   urea 6.2
creat 84

ECG
Normal sinus rhythm

Plan
Surgery tomorrow

Claire Rhodes
Claire Rhodes (FY1 Surgery)

5 September 12:00

Operation Note: Parathyroidectomy
Surgeon: Fraser
Anaesthetist: Stecklenberg (GA)
Assistant: Potter

Procedure:
Transverse incision 2 fingerbreadths above suprasternal notch
Platysma divided and flaps raised
Middle thyroid veins ligated and thyroid gland rotated
Recurrent laryngeal nerves identified and avoided
R and L superior glands removed
R inferior gland removed
½ of L inferior gland removed
Haemostasis
Platysma closed with 2/0 Vicryl
Clips

Postop
Home tomorrow
Check Ca
Clips out 7/7
6/52 follow up in SJF clinic

Simon Fraser
S J Fraser (Consultant Surgeon)

5 September 17:00

WR Miss Potter (ST5)
Sore throat but voice OK
Wound OK; no swelling
Obs fine; pulse 80 BP 136/72 sats 97% (air) RR 14
Can eat/drink
Check bloods tomorrow

Claire Rhodes
Claire Rhodes (FY1 Surgery)

6 September 06:00

Core Trainee O/C: Singh
ATSP by nurses
c/o tingling around mouth and pins and needles in fingers
v anxious
pulse 110 BP 156/90 RR 34
wound fine, no haematoma
chest clear
repeat bloods
ECG

RS
R. Singh (CT1)

6 September 07:00

Bloods

Hb 116	Ca (adj) 1.8	Na 140
WCC 10.3	Alb 34	K 4.1
Plt 126	urea 8.4	
creat 72		

What will you do now?

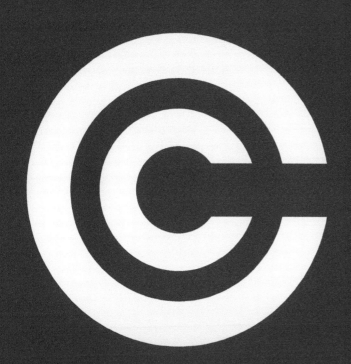

2.9.3

Case 4

4 September 13:00

ITU Discharge Summary

Name	Paulina Petrovka
Case Note Number	4623457
Consultant	Mr Dunn
Summary of admission	This 67-year old woman was admitted to the ITU on 30/08 following an emergency laparotomy for adhesiolysis to relieve small bowel obstruction. She is making a good recovery and can now be discharged back to the ward. She has a nasogastric tube in situ which has been left on free drainage on the advice of Mr Dunn. She has an epidural in situ (bupivacaine/fentanyl) and a urinary catheter.
Medical history	COPD with exercise tolerance of 100 metres Hypertension – on bendroflumethiazide CVA (1999) – on aspirin/atorvastatin Laparotomy for duodenal ulcer (1972) Smoker – 10 cpd NKDA
Cardiac	Pulse 90 (SR), BP 120/84 No inotropic support required during admission
Respiratory	2 L oxygen via nasal cannula Sats 94%
Renal	Urine output 40 mL/h Na 140, K 3.5, urea 8, creat 92
GIT	Nasogastric tube on free drainage: 400 mL last 24 h No bowel movement since surgery
Microbiology	WCC 14.5 neut 10.3 Had prophylactic antibiotics
Neurology	GCS 15 Alert and orientated

4 September 17:00

WR Mr Dunn
Day 5 post laparotomy for adhesiolysis
NGT: 200 mL last 4 h
Leave on free drainage for now
Sips for comfort

Polly Simpson
Polly Simpson (FY1 Surgery)

---

5 September 09:00

<u>WR Miss Abouda (ST3)</u>
NGT: 400 mL overnight
Urine output: 540 mL overnight
Abdomen soft/tender around incision

Polly Simpson
Polly Simpson (FY1 Surgery)

---

5 September 17:00

<u>WR Miss Abouda (ST3)</u>
NGT: 450 mL through the day
Still no flatus – Rx as ileus
Continue IVI

Polly Simpson
Polly Simpson (FY1 Surgery)

---

6 September 08:00

<u>WR Miss Abouda (ST3)</u>
Day 7 post laparotomy
Pulse 80, BP 150/78, afebrile
NGT: 1.8 L last 24 h (950 mL overnight) – Leave on free drainage
Urine output: 620 mL overnight
Abdomen soft but tender
Repeat bloods

Polly Simpson
Polly Simpson (FY1 Surgery)

<u>Bloods</u>

WCC 13.4	Na 139	Lactate 1.6
Hb 92	K 2.9	Mg 0.52
Plt 257	Creat 87	CRP 90
neut 10.2	Urea 9	

What is your role at this stage?

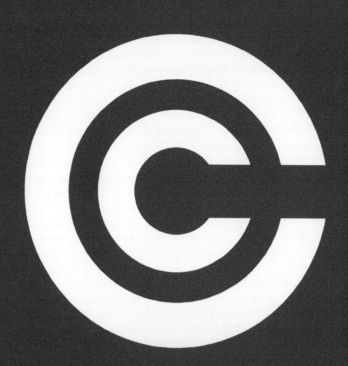

2.9.4

Case 5

5 September 07:00

K Petrov: Surgical CT2 On Call
47yr old ♂ A&E Referral
3/7 h/o progressive L sided facial weakness assd with green, offensive discharge from L ear
Long Hx of problems with L ear since → recurrent infections over past 12/12 requiring PO abx
↑ pain/itching in L ear over past 2/52 → has ENT appt next week
No upper/lower limb neurological symptoms
Swallowing OK

PMHx
HIV +ve: on single-tablet regimen (Atripla)
Borderline DM: diet-controlled
Smokes 10 cpd
Allergic to penicillin → rash and facial swelling

O/E
Temp 37.6°C, Pulse 90, BP 145/95
HS N, Chest clear
Inflamed L ear with pus seen at L EAM
Tenderness around L ear and over mastoid
Otoscopy: R → NAD/L → Inflamed with fleshy lesion at base of canal ?granuloma
Asymmetry of face with L sided facial droop/↓ forehead wrinkling on L with weak eye closure
R CN 7 intact
CNs 1 to 6 and 8 to 12 intact
No other neurology/No e/o meningism

Impression
L facial N palsy
? Recurrent otitis externa

Plan
IV access and bloods (inc. cultures)
Pus swab from ear → M/C/S
Antibiotics
D/w ENT (?r/v in OP clinic today)

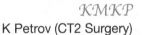
KMKP
K Petrov (CT2 Surgery)

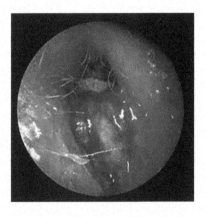

Make a management plan

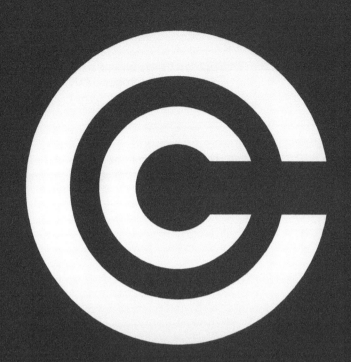

2.9.5

Case 6

6 September 08:00

<u>Case conference with family (mother and father) & Sister Rhodes</u>
24 year old ♂
Day 35 post laparotomy and adhesiolysis for small bowel obstruction.
Background of cerebral palsy and PEG feeding for dysphagia.
Persistently high PEG aspirates and Hickman line in place for TPN.
CT scan with contrast 2 weeks ago showed no sign of mechanical obstruction.

Yesterday's blood results

Hb 115	Na 135	Bili 17
WCC 9.6	K 4.1	ALP 48
Plt 158	Urea 7.0	Alb 24
Creat 62	Mg 0.9	

CT scan performed yesterday demonstrated dilated loops of small bowel but no mechanical cut-off

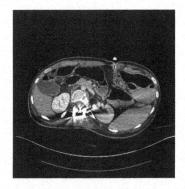 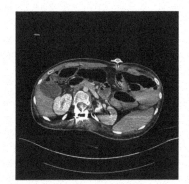

Patient's parents want to take their son home; they already have a package of care in place from before he was admitted. They feel that he is not progressing and could be managed just as well in a familiar environment.

J Jones
Julia Jones (SpR Surgery)

What information do you need before you talk to the family?

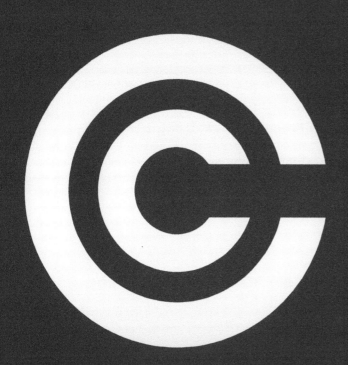

2.9.6

Case 7

4 September 18:00

Miss Evans (ST7 Surgery)
A&E Referral
84yr old ♂ with tender swelling L groin for 2/7
No vomiting but nauseated
No abdominal distension or abdominal pain
Bowels opened yesterday

PMHx
CVA x 2, MI x 1, COPD
Exercise tolerance: 10 yards

SHx
Lives with wife
Retired teacher
Ex smoker

O/E

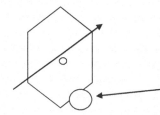

No abdominal tenderness

Tender, irreducible L inguinal hernia / hot / red

No L femoral hernia or R groin hernia

Plan (as d/w Mr Nazir, Consultant O/C) for repair of LIH under local anaesthetic tonight

TRE
Tamsin Evans (ST7 Surgery)

4 September 21:00

Surgeon: Miss T Evans

Operation Note: Open Repair of Left Inguinal Hernia
Local anaesthetic: 30mL 0.5% chirocaine
Antibiotics: Co-amoxiclav 1.2g
Incision: Oblique L groin
Findings: Incarcerated L indirect inguinal hernia (containing viable small bowel)
Procedure: Inguinal canal enetered. Small bowel reduced through the deep ring and the excess sac was excised. A Prolene mesh was shaped to size and secured in place with 2/0 Prolene.
Closure: External oblique: 0 Vicryl
           Scarpa's fascia: 2/0 Vicryl
           Subcuticular 3/0 Monocryl
Post Op: Routine care on ward
           Observe for urinary retention
           Mobilise

TRE
Tamsin Evans (ST7 Surgery)

---

5 September 08:00

<u>WR Mr Nazir</u>
Open repair of LIH last night under LA – wound fine/passing urine
Feeling a bit SOB
ECG: nil acute   CXR: hyperinflated lungs but no consolidation
Needs ABG

Peter Chiu
Peter Chiu (FY1 Surgery)

<u>ABG (on 6L O_2)</u>
pH   7.35
pO_2 9.4
pCO_2 7.2
HCO_3 38
Lactate   1.3
BE   2
Sats   96%

Peter Chiu
Peter Chiu (FY1 Surgery)

---

6 September 8:00

<u>WR Miss Evans</u>
Drowsy: pulse 86, BP 126/82, sats 91% on 6L O_2
Repeat ABG:
pH   7.15
pO_2 7.9
pCO_2 8.9
HCO_3 34
Lactate   1.1
BE   0
Sats   92%

Peter Chiu
Peter Chiu (FY1 Surgery)

What do you need to do now?

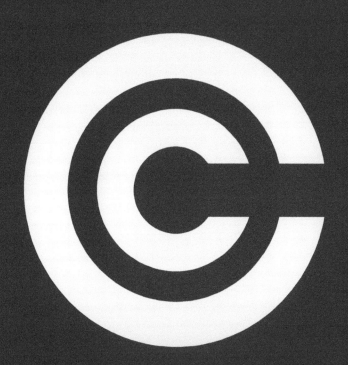

2.9.7

Case 8

4 September 10:30

Angus McAndrew (SpR, General Surgery)
38 yo ♀ admitted with severe central/upper abdominal pain of 5 h in duration. No associated vomiting, some belching. Bowels not opened since the onset of pain. No urinary symptoms and periods have been normal, with no recent discharge or bleeding.
Drug history: chlorpromazine, co-codamol, multivitamins. No allergies.
Past history of schizophrenia/alcohol abuse/pancreatitis (3 x previous US scans in last 4 years have shown no gallstones)
Known IVDU
Lives in a squat with friends and admits to smoking 30/day.
Examination revealed a strange affect, but patient not obviously uncomfortable in the bed.
Nicotine-stained hair and discoloured teeth, but tongue moist and not coated. P86 and regular, BP 130/70.

No abnormal masses
Moves normally with breathing
Voluntary guarding all areas
No peritonism and bowel sounds normal.
Pitted scarring in both groins, but no tenderness or abnormal swelling. Pulses normal.

Plan:
For FBC, U&E, LFT, Amylase, urine dipstick, betaHCG and erect chest X-ray.
Oral clear fluids and attempt IVI
For 10mg morphine IM 4–6 hourly prn

McAndrew
A McAndrew (SpR)

4 September 17.30

V Keen, FY1 in Surgery
Reviewed on evening ward round: still complaining of pain and wanting analgesia ('only morphine works')
No change in clinical status; abdomen still tender but soft
Results: Hb 125, WCC 5.8, Plts 239
Na 143, K 4.8, HCO_3 25, Ur5.5, Cr 77, Alb 34, Ca(corr) 2.15
Amylase 56 LFT N
Urine pH 6.0, else NAD
Pregnancy test negative
CXR clear lungfields and no gas under the diaphragm.

V Keen
Dr Victor Keen (FY1 in Surgery)

What can you do to resolve this situation?

D/W Mr McAndrew (who is still in theatre) for a CT scan of abdomen.

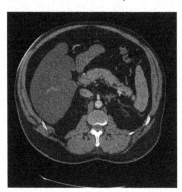

---

5 September 08.00

WR McAndrew
CT shows minor pancreatic calcification, but no other abnormality.
Patient still complaining of pain but she has been leaving the ward frequently through the evening and night. When asked to remain for observations she was openly abusive to members of the nursing ward staff. Requesting larger doses of analgesia for the pain.
Observations stable: pulse 84, BP 118/76, sats 97% on air, RR18
Abdomen soft with epigastric tenderness
Eat/drink as tolerated

V Keen
Dr Victor Keen (FY1 in Surgery)

---

5 September 18:00

FY1 Keen
Patient not at her bed
No observations recorded since this morning

V Keen
Dr Victor Keen (FY1 in Surgery)

---

6 September 08:30

WR McAndrew
Patient returned at 1am eating a takeaway & demanding morphine
Refused all observations overnight and now refusing to engage with us on the WR. Says she has been 'treated worse than an animal'.

V Keen
Dr Victor Keen (FY1 in Surgery)

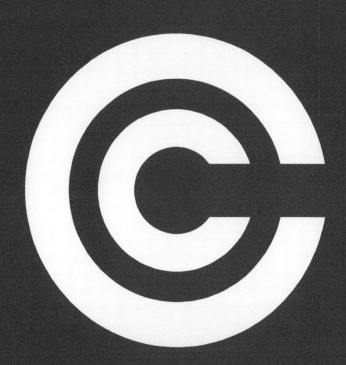

2.9.8

Case 9

5 September 12:00

<u>Tony Di Matteo: Surgical CT O/C</u>
87yr old ♀ c abdominal pain and vomiting
NBO for 1/52
Has not passed flatus for 2/7
Progressive abdominal distension last 2/7
Vomiting +++ today (brown)
Colicky abdominal pain
No prior change in bowel habit
No previous abdominal surgery
Increasingly lethargic last 3/12

<u>PMHx   SHx</u>
HTN – amlodipine   Lives alone in own home
Gout – allopurinol   Needs help c shopping
Ø MI, Ø CVA, Ø DM   Non smoker/No alcohol

<u>O/E</u>
Pulse 110 BP 106/64 Looks dehydrated
HS normal, Chest clear, Sats 96% on air, RR 20

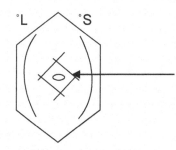

Distended, tympanitic abdomen

Central tenderness but no peritonism

DRE: Collapsed rectum / no mass

<u>Impression</u>
Bowel obstruction

<u>Plan</u>
IV access/Bloods
IV fluids
NGT
Urinary catheter
AXR

Tony Di Matteo
T. Di Matteo (CT2)

<u>Bloods</u>
WCC 12.5 (neut 9.6)   Na 146   Alk Phos 104
Hb 98   K 3.9   ALT 67
Plt 121   Creat 142   Bili 18
Coag N   Urea 13   Alb 30

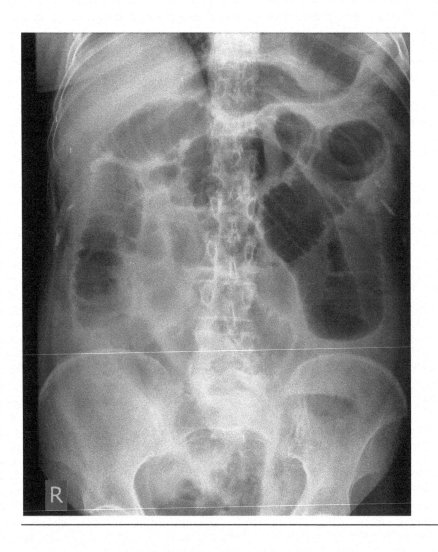

5 September 16:00

<u>WR Mr Fisher (Consultant Surgeon)</u>
Hx suggests bowel obstruction
Abdomen mildly tender
AXR: Dilated loops of small bowel
NGT on free drainage
IVI to maintain urine output >30mL/h
Needs CT scan & repeat bloods in am

PL
Paul Lewis (FY1Surgery)

5 September 19:00

<u>Lewis: FY1 Surgery</u>
CT report from Radiology Consultant: Obstructing distal ascending colonic lesion (suspicious for malignancy) with incompetent ileocaecal valve. Proximal ascending colon is dilated to 7cm while the small bowel is dilated to 4cm. No size significant lymphadenopathy or evidence of metastatic disease.

PL
Paul Lewis (FY1Surgery)

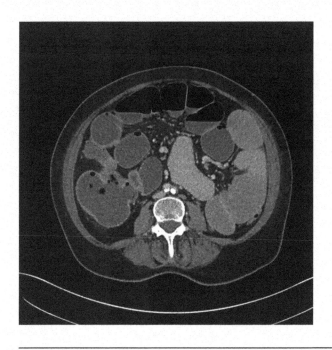

6 September 07:30

Bloods
WCC 11.5 (neut 8.6)   Na 142   Alk Phos 98
Hb 96   K 4.3   ALT 66
Plt 118   Creat 110   Bili 19
Coag N   Urea 10.3   Alb 31

SSK
Sarah King

What is your role in the patient's management at this stage?

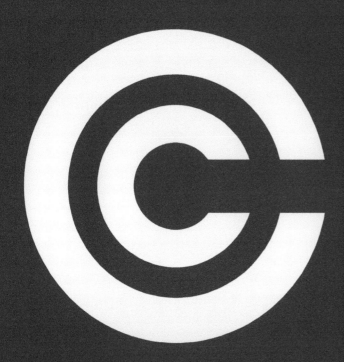

2.9.9

Case 10

5 September 07:45

A De Silva: Surgical CT1

58 yr old ♂

Background: IHD → worsening angina/PVD → R calf claudication 200 yards (R SFA occlusion)/ smoker (20cpd)

Emergency transfer from Cardiology with swollen L arm

Had coronary angiogram yesterday afternoon (via L brachial): 2 x stents inserted

Prescribed dual anti-platelets (aspirin & clopidogrel)

C/o swelling in L ACF post-procedure; seen by Medical FY1 @ 10pm → full range of movement L upper limb → analgesia/elevation/pressure

Swelling increased overnight/awoke @6am c severe pain in L ACF/forearm → seen by Medical CT → skin viable but swollen, tender, erythematous → transferred to SAU

Now has expansile mass in L ACF & pain/tenderness +++ in volar aspect L forearm

Decreased sensation L thumb, 2nd/3rd fingers

Decreased range of movement at L wrist (v. painful)

Good L radial pulse, CRT 1–2s in L fingers

Impression

? post-angiogram bleed

Plan

IV access R arm → bloods/10mg IV morphine

Ultrasound scan L ACF (d/w Radiology SpR – will do on SAU)

A De Silva
A De Silva Bleep 327

What do you need to do to progress this patient's management?

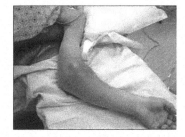

John Conneely

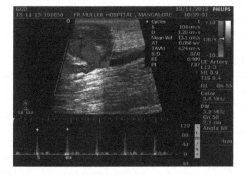

Dr. Rishi Philip Mathew